The Pediatric Patient:

AN APPROACH TO HISTORY AND

PHYSICAL EXAMINATION

The Pediatric Patient

AN APPROACH TO HISTORY AND

PHYSICAL EXAMINATION

PAULA S. ALGRANATI, MD

Assistant Professor
Department of Pediatrics
University of Connecticut Health Center
Farmington, Connecticut

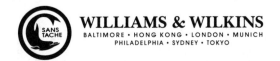

WILLIAMS & WILKINS
BALTIMORE · HONG KONG · LONDON · MUNICH
PHILADELPHIA · SYDNEY · TOKYO

Editor: Timothy S. Satterfield
Associate Editor: Linda Napora
Copy Editor: Mary Kidd
Designer: Karen S. Klinedinst
Illustration Planner: Wayne Hubbel
Production Coordinator: Charles E. Zeller

Accurate indications, adverse reactions, and dosage schedules for drugs are provided in this book, but it is possible that they may change. The reader is urged to review the package information data of the manufacturers of the medications mentioned.

Printed in the United States of America

Library of Congress Cataloging in Publication Data

Algranati, Paula S.
　　The Pediatric Patient: An Approach to History and Physical Examination / Paula S. Algranati.
　　　　p.　　cm.
　　Includes bibliographical references and index.
　　ISBN 0-683-00073-X
　　1. Children—Medical examinations.　2. Physical diagnosis.　3. Medical history taking.　I. Title.
　　[DNLM: 1. Medical History Taking—in adolescence.　2. Medical History Taking—in infancy & childhood.　3. Medical History Taking—methods.　4. Physical Examination—in adolescence.　5. Physical Examination—in infancy & childhood.　6. Physical Examination—methods.　WB 290 A396p]
　　RJ50.A43　1992
　　618.92'007'51—dc20
　　DNLM/DLC
　　for Library of Congress　　　　　　　　　　　　　　　　　　　　91-39788
　　　　　　　　　　　　　　　　　　　　　　　　　　　　　　　　　　CIP

92　93　94　95　96
1　2　3　4　5　6　7　8　9　10

To Bar, Char, and Em

with love forever

Preface

Clinical interactions with children demand special expertise. The purpose of this book is to provide you with the basic skills and knowledge required to succeed within the pediatric setting. The material is presented at a level which assumes mastery of basic history and physical examination in adults. These fundamentals will not be repeated. For example, you have already practiced obtaining a "history of present illness;" you have also practiced auscultating the heart and lungs. This text will teach you how to apply that knowledge to pediatrics. Upon completion, you will be able to obtain age-specific histories and examine children at each developmental stage. You will recognize the equipment in the normal newborn nursery and be able to locate the written information required for the perinatal history. You will identify common congenital anomalies, as well as engage a toddler in play.

This book gives you a place to begin. It is an adjunct to your textbook of pediatrics. It does not contain lists of differential diagnoses of signs or symptoms. That would only obscure more important issues at this stage of your training. By reading this text early in your pediatric experience, you will have the tools to move ahead quickly in learning the more substantive material of pediatrics.

Two assumptions in this book require specific mention. The first is that this text emphasizes findings in the healthy child. Variations of normal and commonly encountered pathology have been added as a second "layer" on the foundation. The emphasis on "normal" is deliberate; it reflects the author's prejudice about the field of pediatrics and the logical way to go about learning it's content. Most children are healthy. If you want to learn about children, it makes sense to begin with what you are most likely to encounter. In addition, a study of normalcy should always precede a study of pathology.

The second assumption relates to the issue of gender. Except for specific discussions about gender-related findings or problems, "he" and "she" are used interchangeably throughout this text. This avoids the necessity of using the more cumbersome "he/she" in every sentence.

This is a "personal book" written from me, to you. Read the illustrative cases and answer the quizzes. My "asides" are intended to remind you to enjoy yourself while learning and practicing!

Acknowledgments

I am particularly indebted to two individuals. During the past seven years, Dr. Paul H. Dworkin has been my colleague, mentor, and friend. He has profoundly influenced my academic pursuits, especially in the areas of medical and health education. Throughout the development of this text, he has provided advice and encouragement, as well as a painstaking review of the entire manuscript. His continued guidance and friendship are cherished. My husband, Dr. Barry Izenstein, has provided unlimited love, companionship, and enthusiasm. He is truly a partner in every endeavor and encourages me to flourish within multiple roles simultaneously. On numerous occasions he has been both mother and father so that I could continue writing without interruption. To him I am indebted beyond words.

I am grateful to my colleagues who have critically reviewed chapters of the book and offered many helpful suggestions: Drs. Michael D. Bailie, Leon Chameides, Donald Hight, Carol R. Leicher, Vicki Levander, Richard Luftman, Chris Nusbacher, Susan K. Ratzan, Ted S. Rosenkrantz, Nadine Wenner, and Steven Wenner. In addition, I thank my other colleagues in the Department of Pediatrics at the University of Connecticut Health Center who have served as important resources, never hesitating when I asked for assistance. Dr. Bailie, former chairman of the Department of Pediatrics, deserves special mention. He provided the opportunity and the atmosphere to pursue my interest in clinical skills education and in ambulatory pediatrics as well.

The text is immeasurably enhanced by the photographs of Gregory Kriss. He displayed infinite kindness and patience with our models. I am pleased to have worked with Joyce Lavery, who skillfully provided the illustrations. I am grateful to Drs. Henry M. Feder, Jr., Stanley F. Glazer, Robert M. Greenstein, Douglas H. MacGilpin, and Arthur M. Sher, who willingly shared their extensive slide collections. I am particularly indebted to Dr. Sidney Hurwitz, who so cheerfully and generously offered whatever I needed from his well-known collection of dermatologic photographs. I also thank Dale Hogan for so ably typing many versions of the manuscript.

I acknowledge the important influence of Dr. Richard Solomon in the development of this text. I was inspired by his curricular material on "making friends," in which a developmentally oriented approach to interacting with pediatric patients is taught. The book is sprinkled with examples that reflect this material.

Joan Parker, my friend and first editor, was responsible for the conception of this project. Throughout, she cajoled, convinced, and commiserated, providing enthusiasm and thoughtful guidance.

The editors and staff at Williams & Wilkins have been exceedingly helpful. In particular, I thank John Gardner and Michael Fisher for their enthusiasm about my writing, and Tim Satterfield for his continued support of my efforts.

My women friends are especially cherished. Rather than leave anyone out, I thank them collectively for continuously touching base, checking in, and being there.

Throughout these past years my children, Emily and Charlie, have thrived and flourished in no small part due to their "other mother," Sandra Lasseter. Without her, this book would not have been completed.

Finally, as always, I am thankful for the unqualified love and enthusiasm provided by my parents, Dorothy and Ralph Algranati. Their life-long encouragement and support have empowered and sustained me.

Contents

CHAPTER 1

Introduction

HOW TO USE THIS BOOK

Begin by reading this chapter. It contains some general principles of pediatric physical diagnosis. It will introduce you to the settings in which you will be working. It also supplies guidelines to follow in determining the type and quantity of information you need to acquire in different encounters. Finally, it reviews the special concepts and techniques of measurement unique to pediatric medicine.

The rest of the book is written in chronologic order. The first part of each chapter describes the interval history and physical exam relevant to a particular age group. At the end of each chapter, an illustrative case is presented for reinforcement. The cases also present concepts which may be applied to problem solving.

The appendix contains tables that you will use when examining children (e.g., growth charts, vital signs, Tanner stages). It also contains an outline of the comprehensive pediatric history and physical. This outline may prove useful in select instances in which a detailed history and physical exam may be indicated.

Students reading this book for the first time will find it easiest to read from beginning to end. That way, you build upon information in sequence and avoid needing repetition. For example: the mother of a three-year-old might ask you why her daughter's feet turn in when she walks. The explanation for this might be related to the hip, leg, or foot exam. Close examination of these body parts for congenital anomalies are integral parts of the newborn and infant exams. The descriptions of these are introduced in those chapters where they first apply. By the time you reach the toddler chapter, you will know most of the maneuvers necessary to answer her question. The final maneuver, defining normal gait, will be described at that time.

THE SETTINGS

The Nursery

Student Tasks

1. Recognize the equipment in the newborn nursery.

2. Locate the written information required for the pre-and perinatal history.

The nursery may be the site of your very first clinical encounter with children. As you step into the room, undoubtedly someone will stop you and say, "Did you scrub?" Don't be put off. Find a sink (there will be one right outside). After removing your watch and other jewelry except your rings, wash your hands and forearms vigorously with the liquid soap or soap-impregnated sponge for approximately three minutes. Dry off with a paper towel, put on an overgown, and try walking in again. One more thing: leave your stethoscope outside. Borrow one from the nursery (this will have a small diaphragm), and wash the diaphragm off with an alcohol wipe. This is a good time to gather the other equipment you'll need: a paper tape measure, a nursery otoscope-ophthalmoscope kit, a watch with a second hand (there may be a clock on the wall), and a tongue blade.

Take a look around. You will see swaddled babies in open bassinets, (Figure 1.1) lying on their sides or abdomens. Swaddling calms babies, and the belly-down position prevents aspiration of feeds.

There will be a few babies under overhead radiant warmers (Figure. 1.2). These babies are "brand new," having recently come from the delivery room. The heat generated from above is regulated in response to a temperature probe that is taped to the baby's skin. Babies are kept under the warmer until their own temperature has achieved stability in a normal range. Achieving stability may take several hours or just a few minutes. Smaller babies and sick babies have more difficulty than healthy term infants in achieving and maintaining a stable temperature.

Babies who require prolonged ambient temperature control are placed in incubators. The incubator has portholes which open. These allow you to put your arms through, in order to examine, feed, or change a baby without loss of heat. Internal ambient temperature is automatically regulated. Occasionally there will be a plastic hood (attached to an oxygen source) covering the baby's head. If you need total access to the baby in an incubator, one entire side opens up.

You may also see a panel of fluorescent bulbs or a spot light directed at a jaundiced

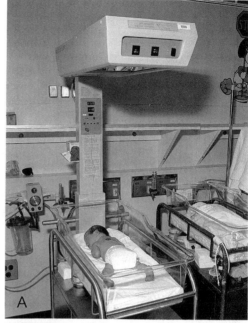

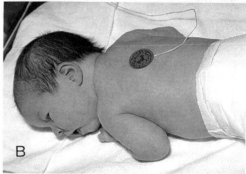

Figure 1.2.   Overhead warmer.
Figure 1.2A. The baby is closely observed during the transitional period after birth.
Figure 1.2B. Heat generated from above is regulated in response to a temperature probe that is taped to the baby's skin.

infant (Figure 1.3). Phototherapy converts bilirubin to water-soluble photoisomers which can be eliminated by the baby. A baby "under lights" will be wearing "sunglasses" (eye patches) for protection from potential retinal damage (documented in animals only).

Other, more sophisticated apparatuses, such as cardiac monitors, apnea monitors, i.v. set-ups, etc., may also be found in some "normal" newborn nurseries. During your

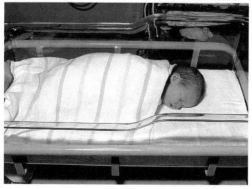

Figure 1.1.   Open bassinet. The stable newborn is swaddled and placed on side or abdomen.

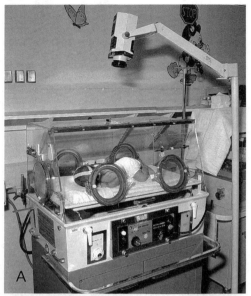

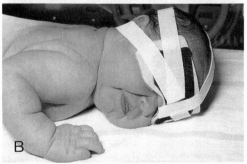

Figure 1.3A. Photography light is directed at infant inside incubator.
Figure 1.3B. During phototherapy, the eyes are covered for protection against potential retinal damage.

physical diagnosis courses and introductory pediatrics rotations, it is unlikely that you will be examining babies attached to these machines on a routine basis.

Information about a baby you are interested in may be found in several places. There may be a formal chart in a chart rack. This may contain a copy of the mother's delivery sheet. This is usually filled out by the obstetrician at the time of delivery. Portions of the prenatal history will be included. You may also find the footprint sheet. This will contain birth weight and length. Be sure and look for nurses' notes. These contain valuable information about

the birth and often also contain some details of psycho-social history. In addition, there are daily nurses' notes written about each infant. These may be in the chart, on a clip board by the crib, or on one master clip board containing information about all the babies in the nursery. Expect these to contain daily weights, feeding patterns, elimination records (voiding and stooling), and comments about problems such as jaundice. Finally, don't hesitate to go out to the obstetrics floor and ask to see the mother's chart, too. This will expand upon the prenatal history and often contains vital information. Sometimes this information will not surface during your discussions with the mother either because she doesn't quite understand exactly what occurred, doesn't remember it, or doesn't choose to share it with you.

Read all available information about a baby before you examine her. This knowledge will guide your exam. It will make "gestational aging" easier; it may point towards a search for specific anomalies or clue you into concerns that mom will address with you when you interview her. It is not "cheating" to have this information first.

In the newborn chapter, we will review the specifics of the prenatal history that you will obtain from the mother. After looking over the baby's (and if necessary, the mother's) chart you must decide whether to examine her infant or interview her first. In practice, we often examine the baby first and fill in the remaining details with mom later. We do it this way because it saves time, and the records available to us answer most of our questions. But the most important reason is to be able to immediately answer mom's first question when you meet her. That question will be, "Is my baby normal?"

Once you've gained some confidence, you might want to try another approach: examine the baby at the mom's bedside. It's always nice for parents to observe a newborn exam, because it allows them to ask questions as you procede. Variations within normal findings can be pointed-out and discussed, dispelling early concerns. Many pediatricians feel this is really the ideal way to approach the first exam. However, at this point, most of you will not feel prepared to do this. That's okay. It's a model you may want to follow in the future, when you're more confident about your abilities.

The Office

Student Task

1. Distinguish between the outpatient encounters which require a comprehensive history and physical exam vs. those in which an interval history and/or focused physical exam may suffice.

You may be encountering children in outpatient settings for a variety of reasons: well child care, illness visits, and diagnostic consultations. These might take place in medical centers or free-standing clinics, emergency rooms, or private offices. In your introductory courses, you have spent many hours practicing on patients using the comprehensive history and physical format. In the ambulatory setting, it is not always appropriate to use this. Students often have difficulty in making the transition to situations in which an interval history or focused physical exam is required. Below are some guidelines to follow in the various clinical situations you will encounter in the outpatient setting.

1. Before you enter the room, ask the nurse if this is a "new" or an "old" patient to the practice or institution and what the stated reason for the visit is. If that is impossible, ask the parent very early in the encounter for the specific reason for the visit. That way, your history taking will be more efficient. Parents frequently have several problems in mind. We will speak further about multiple agendas in describing the interview.

2. If the patient is an **established one,** review the chart before you enter, keeping the reason for the visit in mind. Glance at previous well child visits and problem visits (particularly the most recent visits) to high-light ongoing issues. If there is a problem list, review this carefully. The outpatient chart may also contain information about immunizations, medicines, and allergies, as well as family and social history. In other words, it should provide all the parts of the complete history up until "now" for you. Before you begin the encounter, review all the sections which might be relevant to this visit.

If this is a **well child visit,** consult the age-appropriate flow sheet provided in each chapter to guide your history. Some practices use flow sheets that you can follow, right within the patient's chart. Chart review will highlight resolved and ongoing health maintenance problems.

If this is a **problem visit,** follow the rules you have learned on adult patients in pursuing such information as duration, severity, and associated symptoms, etc. Chart review will clarify previous diagnostic and therapeutic maneuvers; it may also contain plans for managing recurrences. Sometimes, the age-appropriate flow sheet will be of assistance in dealing with a particular problem (e.g., to remind you about normal behavior). Remember to ask if the patient has received care for this problem somewhere else, too.

3. Sometimes you will see patients who are **unfamiliar** to the staff of the facility where you are working. This commonly occurs in a busy practice, emergency room, or consultative facility. Before you enter the examining room, make sure there really isn't an old chart hiding in medical records. (This happens in the emergency room frequently.) The extent to which you will need to obtain a comprehensive history on a **"new"** patient will be determined by the nature of the visit and the age of the patient. If the patient's family has carried old records with them, review these thoroughly before beginning your formal history. For routine information (immunizations, birth statistics, etc.), you can usually rely on what's written down. For complicated problems, take the history again. Too often, some crucial piece of

information has been overlooked or discarded. Your job is to find answers that haven't yet surfaced, and you can only do that by taking a fresh look.

New patients for well child care, complicated problems, or second opinions always require a comprehensive history. The age-appropriate flow sheet may be consulted in addition to obtaining details about current functioning.

If you are working in an emergency room or "walk in" and seeing a new patient for a relatively **routine problem,** ask a few questions to get a general sense about the child's previous state of health. Time constraints will necessitate that you develop the ability to do this briefly. For instance "Has he been pretty healthy up until now?; has he had any major illnesses or injuries in the past?; any surgeries or hospitalizations?; is he currently on any medications or is he being followed for any specific medical problems?; does he have any known allergies?."

The **ill infant under two or three months of age** presents a special challenge. There are usually no short cuts. When this type of child presents to a facility that doesn't know him, it is crucial to obtain a comprehensive history, including the prenatal history.

4. How detailed should your physical exam be? The same rules apply as with histories. It depends on the reason for the visit. **Well child** visits and **complicated problems** always require fairly complete exams. What you emphasize depends on the age of the patient. Use the appropriate chapter in this text to guide you. The completeness of your exam for an **episodic problem** visit is also determined by the reason for the visit. If the complaint is contact dermatitis, you will need to examine all skin surfaces. In an otherwise well-appearing child, this is sufficient. However, if during your initial exam you notice that the child has some unusual bruises (and the possibility of child abuse occurs to you), take a deep breath and obtain further history and physical exam information. This is a good example of when reviewing the chart (before you went in) might have been helpful. If there is no old chart, you need to gather the pertinent information yourself.

The rule for the **ill infant** applies to physical exams, too. Most of the time (e.g., in the presence of fever, irritability, or decreased feeding), nothing less than a complete physical is acceptable.

The Pediatric Ward
Student Tasks

1. Identify the emotional barriers to compliance in the hospitalized child and family.

2. Identify the physical barriers which impede physical exams in the hospitalized child and give examples of how to overcome these impediments.

Most pediatric wards contain children with a potpourri of admission diagnoses. Whatever the reason for admission, an evaluation of a hospitalized child must always begin with a complete history and physical.

It is helpful to remember the great degree of stress experienced by the hospitalized child. He's coping with separation from family and friends. He's forced to adjust to the unfamiliar and frightening environment of the hospital. If he's old enough, he may be worried about his illness and its implications. Therefore, you should expect him to exhibit: fear, anger, regression, and non-compliant or withdrawal behavior. Later on in this text, we will discuss the particular concerns of children at each developmental stage. Using that information while relating to and examining children will be particularly helpful in the stressful setting of the ward.

Parents also experience heightened anxiety when their child is hospitalized. Try to uncover this when you take the history. Ask about the other family members, too. By acknowledging that you "hear" parental concerns, you will begin to form an alliance with them. This will facilitate histories, physicals, and, ultimately, therapeutic plans.

Hospital rooms and hospitalized children (because of the nature of equipment required) have physical barriers which impede physical exams. Most of the time, you can "work around" them. Here are some suggestions:

1. Do as complete an exam as possible. If the child has an i.v., cast, or other limb encumberance, examine all other body parts first. You can certainly walk around the bed or move the bed to get to him. If something is "pinned down" to the bed, (e.g., an i.v. with an arm board) ask the nurse if you can unpin it for the duration of the exam. The arm board is protection for the i.v. and should allow the involved arm to be moved. Just remember to repin it before you leave.

2. Don't be insulted by this next one. Take the crib rails down when you need access to an infant, but don't forget to put them back up when you are ready to leave him.

3. When you have finished examining the child in bed, (if he is old enough) have him get up and walk for you. If you have some doubt about whether he is allowed to do this, ask! It is particularly easy to forget this part of the exam (and miss some important findings). . . . As a medical student, I had the unfortunate experience of examining an adolescent girl who had been transferred to the psychiatric ward from another hospital for treatment of anorexia nervosa and depression. She was so weak that she spent most of her day either in bed or in a wheel chair. When I assisted her in walking, I observed a marked lateral head and body tilt. There was a large brain tumor responsible for all of her signs and symptoms!

4. Don't let the seriously ill child intimidate you. Ask before you start, what can be detached and what can't. For instance, sometimes a monitor can be detached or shut off while you are with the patient. However, some of the time (e.g., a child on a ventilator) there will be an extremely delicate apparatus attached that should not

be tampered with. That doesn't mean that the whole exam should be deferred. You will just not be able to move the patient's head.

5. Uncooperative children may require you to ask for assistance from a parent or nurse. You may need to ask your supervisor if certain parts of the exam are really necessary. (Usually the answer is yes!) . . . Another example of this from my medical school days comes to mind. I was examining a child with a stiff neck who was admitted with the diagnosis of meningitis. She would not cooperate in opening her mouth for a pharyngeal exam. When she was held down and her pharynx became visible, so did her enormous peritonsillar abcess! That was the explanation for her stiff neck.

6. Many children are hospitalized for diagnosis or treatment of infection. Therefore, you might encounter isolation and precaution signs at the entrance to a room or cubicle. Follow the directions on the door and wear the appropriate gowns, gloves, or masks as required. You may also have to use equipment (e.g., a stethoscope) that is left in the room for your patient only. The precautions make a complete exam cumbersome but not impossible. If you use some of your own equipment, remember to cleanse it with alcohol before and after your exam.

7. The same rules apply to comatose children as they do to comatose adults. Coma is a sign, not a diagnosis. Even though a comatose child cannot actively cooperate, you still need to do as complete an exam as possible under the circumstances. If you need to examine a child who is sedated, do all of the parts of the exam except those which require alertness or active cooperation. Come back when he is more alert and complete your exam.

8. Sometimes you will find your patient in the playroom or child life room. First, observe him at play. You may make some useful observations. Then see if you can negotiate him back into his room. Make a judgement as to the necessity of bringing him back at that moment. If you have time, wait until he is done playing. If not, bring a

toy back with you. Don't perform intrusive or painful procedures in the playroom.

THE ENCOUNTER

Each of you can conjure up sights, sounds, and even smells from childhood experiences. Your first pediatric encounters will revive old memories. For some of you, this might be the kindly smile of an old family "doc." For others, it might be a more frightening image. Running away from the office nurse who held the "shot" is still a very vivid picture for me!

You probably also have vague memories of a relatively short conversation between doctor and parent that went something like this, "Well, Mrs. Jones, how has Johnny been? . . . Any problems? . . . Now, let's take a look at him. . . ."

A contemporary conversation might sound like this, "Well, Mr. and Mrs. Jones, how nice to see you. . . . How have you been? . . . What's life like now that there are three of you? . . . How have you managed to work out your schedules with the new baby? . . . What kinds of difficulties have you encountered? . . ."

A second contemporary conversation might go like this, "Well, Ms. Smith, how are things going? . . . How are you managing with your new baby? . . . Who else is living in the house with you? . . . Are you getting any support from the father of the baby? . . ."

Both of these conversations typify how patient encounters have changed. As our patient needs have evolved, so has our approach to child health care. The "check-up" has been replaced with "health care maintenance." As the name has become more complex, so has the concept. There are two reasons for this. The first is that physical ill health has diminished. Perinatal survival, infectious disease prevention, and treatment have all benefited from scientific advances. The second reason is that with the increasing complexity of our society, "social ill health" has become much more prevalent.[2] Single parent families, substance abuse, child abuse, etc., affect an enormous percentage of our patients and their families. Even in the "ideal" situation, parents and children are coping with issues surrounding daycare, maternity leaves, shared home responsibilities, etc. Physicians who take care of children are often the only professionals to monitor on an ongoing basis the impact that these situations are having on our young patients and their families.

Keeping the above discussion in mind, the following are the components of child health maintenance:

1. **Establish a trusting and two-way working relationship with the patient and family.**
2. **Obtain a history to assess physical and developmental progress of your patient. Assess family wellness and the impact of family problems on your patient.**
3. **Perform a physical exam to assess wellness (including growth and development) and pick up hidden problems.**
4. Provide appropriate screening tests and immunizations.
5. Provide anticipatory guidance.
6. Provide diagnostic and therapeutic intervention when necessary.

Components **1, 2,** and **3** are what you should concentrate on for now. It doesn't matter whether you are seeing children as part of your physical diagnosis course or during your formal pediatric clerkship. The basic tasks of the encounter always begin with **1, 2,** and **3.**

Components 4, 5, and 6 will be emphasized during your clinical rotations, once your basic pediatric skills are in place.

The Pediatric History

During pediatric history taking, begin with establishment of a trusting and two-way working relationship with the patient and the family. By obtaining a history, you begin the assessment of the physical and developmental progress of your patient. You also begin the assessment of family wellness and the impact of family problems on your patient.

THE "STYLE" OF THE PEDIATRIC HISTORY[3,4]
Student Tasks

1. Identify the historians in pediatric interviews.
2. List some possible hidden agendas in pediatric histories.
3. Explain the techniques of preparation, observation, and modification.

During pediatric interviews, there are at least two "historians" present: parent and child. (The adolescent interview is the exception). The initial history is given second hand. That is, parents will give you their interpretation of the patient's signs and symptoms. If your patient is old enough, ask him for the history, too. Join parents in "looking at the problem" from the child's point of view. Listen to both accounts. While you are listening, remember that long-standing patterns of parent-child interaction have influenced what you are told.

When you listen, sit down! This establishes better eye contact and is less threatening (than when you stand), and conveys the message that you aren't rushing. Don't sit on a high stool either; find a chair of similar height to the one that the parent occupies.

There may be one or more hidden agendas. The parents' agenda might contain unstated fears, guilt, or anger. The child's may reflect underlying fears of bodily harm and the fantasies he has woven with those fears. The chief complaint may only be the "tip of the iceberg." Start each interview with an open-ended question and become more directive later. For example, rather than saying, "So, you think Johnny has another ear infection?", you might open with, "What brought you in to see us today?" Later on, you might ask, "Is there anything else about this situation that's bothering you?" The mother of the child with an ear infection is worried about the source of her child's fever. Perhaps she is also wondering about the effects of the infection on his hearing. Hopefully, you will identify the "real" concerns that lead to the encounter. Try to deal with those feelings in a reassuring and nonjudgmental manner. Recognize that this is an "art" that takes time to acquire.

Remember to give information to your patient as well as to his or her parent. Children hear everything that is said between parent and doctor. They need explanations as well. The specifics of "how" to talk with children will be dealt with throughout the various chapters.

Before you enter the room, review the appropriate history outline (either an age appropriate flow sheet found in the individual chapters, or the comprehensive history outline found in the appendix) and the patient's chart (this is **preparation**). The more you know about your patient's progress and the issues that are likely to be important, the more comfortable you will feel during history taking. Preparation will also enable you to concentrate on making **observations** as you converse. Ultimately you will want to **modify** your questions based upon your observations. When you are able to do this, your history taking will become more meaningful and focused. The technique of using **preparation, observation,** and **modification,** during your pediatric encounters will be reinforced throughout this text.

THE "CONTENT" OF THE PEDIATRIC HISTORY: INTERVAL AND COMPREHENSIVE
Student Tasks

1. List the five major categories of information contained in an age-appropriate interval history.
2. Give examples of questions pertinent to each of the five major categories of the age-appropriate interval history.
3. Review the outline of the comprehensive history in the Appendix of this book.

In each chapter (except the newborn), there are history flow sheets headed by five major categories:

Table 1.1
History Flow Sheet Categories[a]

General Care	Growth and Development	Developmental Milestones	General Health (ROS and PMH)	Family and Psycho-Social

[a]Flow sheets and explanatory notes adapted from Dworkin PH, Wible KL, Sutherland MC, Humphrey N. *Manual of pediatric anticipatory guidance*. Morgantown, West Virginia; West Virginia University Medical Center, 1985.

Learn these headings and their explanations. The specific questions are geared to the age and developmental stage of the child at the time of the encounter. (The newborn chapter outlines the prenatal and perinatal history.)

Explanatory notes follow each set of flow sheets. The notes expand upon and clarify the word cues provided on the flow sheets. Sometimes they offer specific examples of phrasing you may use in your discussions. Each set of explanatory notes deals with an age range (rather than one specific age). This method of organization provides you with a variety of possible issues to discuss under each heading. This is because normal progress through each stage varies from child to child. To clarify how this works, here's an example. On the two-month flow sheet, a "cue word" under General Care . . . Sleep . . . is "methods used." It is appropriate to ask if the parents have any special routines (e.g., rocking or walking with their infant) at bedtime. On the four-month flow sheet, a "cue word" under General Care . . . Sleep . . . is "own room." At the four-month visit, it is appropriate to ask if the infant sleeps in his own room. By age two months, many infants are already sleeping in their own rooms (while some infants never do). By reading the explanatory notes for all of early infancy at one time, you will be aware of how your patient's history may differ (normally) from the specific "cues" on the appropriate chronologic flow sheet. In other words, use the "cues" as starting points to discuss issues, but keep the entire age range in mind as you proceed.

This is the information you would obtain at a **well child visit.** (It updates you since the previous visit.) For a **problem (or illness) visit,** emphasize the content areas related to the problem. For example, a well child visit requires questions about home safety. A problem visit for a toddler's "out of control" behavior will also require discussion about this area; a problem visit for a toddler's immunization reaction will not. **There is no need to follow a definite order in obtaining information. Nor is it necessary to ask about every one of the individual items listed in the specific visits.** As long as you use the general categories as guidelines, you will obtain most of the important information.

If you need to obtain a **comprehensive history,** you should follow the outline of the pediatric comprehensive history found in the Appendix. The information in the comprehensive history is organized slightly differently from that in the age-appropriate interval history. The age-appropriate interval history is really just the "update" of a comprehensive history. As you familiarize yourself with the flow sheets and their explanations, all the components of the pediatric history will become familiar to you. Then, if you need to obtain a comprehensive history, you will be able to follow the outline in the Appendix with greater understanding of the various components.

Remember to begin with a general, open-ended question. The parent or patient will tell you what problem areas need to be concentrated on. During the physical exam, it is very unusual for a "surprise" to arise. That is, one rarely finds a significant problem in the physical exam without having had some clue beforehand from the history.

General Care

This type of information refers to activities that make up a child's day. The content includes eating, sleeping, and elimination patterns. It also refers to tasks that parents perform in order to care for a child such as accident prevention, cleansing methods, etc. **If you have time, you might even ask the parent or child (if they are old enough) to describe a typical day.** This method often gives answers when specific questions did not.

Growth and Development

This category of information refers to questions about the three major lines of development: affective development, cognitive development, and physical development.[5] As you begin to gather this history, use simultaneous "observation" to confirm or modify what you are told.

Affective development refers to emotional and behavioral development. Questions in this area relate to phenomenon such as: *synchrony* (responses between an infant and caretaker), *temperament* (behavioral style), *attachment* (the establishment of a unique relationship between infant and caretaker), and *autonomy-independence* (the process of separating from parents and establishing a separate identity). Other questions in this area will focus on: *impulse control* (the child's ability to self regulate his behavior), *gender identity* (the child's definition of himself/herself as a boy or girl), *peer interaction* (the way in which the child relates to his peers), and *adolescence* (the child's progress through the various "tasks" of adolescence). **Asking a parent to describe, "What kind of baby (or child) is he?" will introduce the subject of affective development.**

Cognitive development refers to the development of intellect. According to Piaget, a child evolves through four major stages of cognitive development.[6] These are *sensory-motor intelligence* (the infant explores the environment using his sensory and motor tools such as feeling, seeing, and hearing); *pre-operational intelligence* (approximate ages 2–7) the child begins to use meaningful language and representational thought (e.g., when words symbolize objects or people); *concrete operations* (approximately ages 7–

11) the child's capacity to conceptualize objects, people, or events becomes more sophisticated (e.g., he views things as parts of larger systems; he can "order" things, use logic, and understand different points of view) and *formal operations* (the most advanced level of thought which begins in adolescence and continues into the late teens (e.g., the child can now use abstract reasoning and test hypotheses)).[7] The content of questions in the area of cognitive development will relate to such items as *language acquisition, reasoning ability, school readiness,* and *career plans* (e.g., the adolescent becomes capable of thinking about the abstract future and can begin to entertain realistic thoughts about career goals).

Physical development includes descriptions of: *state organization* (transitions in states of consciousness in the infant), *motor development* (progress towards becoming physically autonomous), *growth rate* (this refers to normal periods of rapid, e.g., early infancy and adolescence, and slower, e.g., early school-age growth, as well as abnormal growth), and *puberty* (physical changes during adolescence).

Each flow sheet contains age-appropriate questions about each of these areas of development. The accompanying explanatory notes clarify definitions or offer specific phrasing for questions.

Developmental Milestones

Developmental milestones are abilities achieved by the majority of normal children by certain, predictable ages. Under this heading, you will find questions to ask parents and/or skills to verify during your exam. This information supplements the information obtained in the previous category. Combined, these two categories of information provide informal developmental monitoring of your patient. Information obtained by history includes parental interpretation (and therefore, possible bias), and the results must be viewed with caution. If you find a possible problem (when a child consistently lags behind the expected norm) then more formal screening or testing may be appropriate.

Many pediatricians routinely perform a more formal developmental screen on all their patients, such as the Denver Developmental Screening Test (DDST) at age one year and the Preschool Readiness Experimental Screening Scale (PRESS) during the school entry physical examination, to supplement the informal questions at interval visits. A copy of the newly revised "Denver" (Denver II) will be found in the appendix of this book. Correct use and interpretation of this screening instrument requires specific training which is beyond the scope of this book. It has been made available to you in case you will be trained to use it during your pediatrics rotation.

General Health

This category highlights recent or chronic medical problems experienced by your patient. It includes an update on **Past Medical History** (PMH) and **Review of Systems** (ROS). Refer to the individual flow sheets for the most important age-appropriate topics. For a more comprehensive review of past medical history and review of systems refer to the Appendix (Comprehensive History).

This is the time to ask the mother of a four-month-old how her baby reacted to her first Diptheria, Tetanus, Pertussis (DTP) injection given at the time of the previous (two-month) visit. Or, if you know (by having read the chart beforehand) that an iron supplement was prescribed at the last visit, this is the time to ask if the toddler has been getting it and if there have been any reactions to it. Third, if the parent mentions that her child had a hearing or vision screen in school, find out what the results were.

Family History—Psycho-Social History

Begin with a general question like, "How are you doing?" . . . "How are you feeling?" . . . "How's everyone else at home doing?" . . . "Are there any problems?"

This category assesses family wellness, both physical and psychosocial. Illness of family members impacts significantly on everyone in the household (as does childhood illness). Also, major life events in the household (such as mother returning to work, parents separating, birth of a new sibling) also impact significantly on all family members. The impact of family problems may be manifested by either physical or behavioral symptoms. Unless you ask specifically about family stresses, this important information may remain obscured.

The Pediatric Physical Exam

An experienced pediatrician is comfortable interacting with children. In addition, at the conclusion of an encounter, he or she has a "sense" of whether or not a child is growing and developing properly. Haven't you wondered how to acquire that comfortable "style" and "gestalt" with pediatric patients? Practice is only part of the answer. The other part comes from knowing how to apply some scientific principles during each exam.

During a pediatric physical examination, continue cementing a trusting and two-way working relationship with the patient and the family. Assess wellness (including growth and development) and pick up hidden problems.

THE "STYLE" OF THE PEDIATRIC PHYSICAL EXAM[1,8,9,10,11]

Student Task

1. List examples of useful modification techniques which improve patient cooperation.

The easiest way to accomplish an accurate and complete physical exam is to secure the cooperation of your patient. Pediatricians are especially proud of their ability to do this. It is important to smile and appear relaxed and approachable. But sometimes, particularly with infants and toddlers, friendly overtures are not enough. Predictable, developmentally-related fears, or previous frightening experiences can ruin a potentially positive clinical encounter before it even begins. How can you maximize your chances of "making friends" with your young patients?[1] (This is another example of a technique you were introduced to earlier)—by **preparation, observation,** and **modification.**

This is the second reason to **review the flow sheet and chart before entering the room.** The "Growth and Development" and "Developmental Milestones" columns will supply you with information to estimate what a child is likely to *understand, enjoy,* and *fear.* The old chart will add specific information *about his or her temperament, achievements, previous medical experiences, and parent-child relationships.*

For example: Carl Davos has arrived for a nine-month health maintenance visit. You notice the Davos family at the measuring station in the hallway. Carl is accompanied by his mother and his six-year-old sister, Carol. Before you walk into the room, review the flow sheet for the nine-month visit and review Carl's past history.

You see that the "Growth and Development" column on the flow sheet for a nine-month-old says, "Attachment: clinging . . . Temperament: predictable responses . . . Cognitive: object permanence and causality." The "Developmental Milestones" column says: "pulls to stand . . . creeps . . . transfers well . . . peek-a-boo." His chart contains no problem visits, and no problems listed on the problem list. Sibling rivalry has not been particularly problematic; in fact, the relationship between the two children has been very positive. Carl's mother has described him as an "easy child."

With the information you now have, you know that Carl probably will: fear being separated from his mother, but will creep around the room if his mother is close by; will understand a game of peek-a-boo (object permanence); will enjoy handling and transferring small objects; will be distracted by his sister.

As you enter the room, use **observation** to confirm and **modify** what you've already predicted. Is your patient: awake, sleeping, crying, laughing, etc.? If this is a "sick" visit,

you should expect that your patient will be crankier and more clingy than usual; if it's at the end of the day, he's likely to be less cooperative, too.

To deter fears, use modification[1]:

1. Avoid predictable conflicts if at all possible (e.g., separating a child from his mother).
2. Alter your body language (voice, gaze, touch) to become as nonthreatening as possible.
3. Maximize a child's cognitive ability and achievements to familiarize him with you and your procedures (e.g., if a child has an appreciation of object permanence, you can play peek-a-boo or play at hiding one of your instruments).
4. Maximize what a child enjoys doing to distract him (e.g., a child who enjoys manipulating small objects may be handed some colorful blocks while you listen to his chest).
5. Avoid repetition of previous frightening medical experiences if at all possible or defer them to the end of the encounter.
6. Make parents your ally (e.g., have the toddler's parent participate in the exam by holding the child in his lap and helping with distraction or play while you proceed).

Let's get back to Carl to see how this all works. At nine months he is beginning to experience separation and stranger anxiety. As you enter the room, he is playing with blocks on the floor with his sister. He glances up at you with a worried look, and begins to creep toward his mother. Keep your distance! Speak softly and make eye contact with a friendly smile towards his mother. His mother picks him up and puts him in her lap. You pull out some small rubber dolls from your pocket and put them in mom's lap, without looking directly at Carl yet. You begin your history taking with mom and also converse with Carl's sister. You are giving Carl time to get used to your presence before direct interaction. Next, pull out some of your instruments, put them on the table in front of Carl and let him feel them and hold them. This gives him the opportunity to familiarize himself with them. He will want to mouth them, so instead offer him a small (not too small) plastic toy that can be cleansed later. When it is time to examine him, don't separate him from mom! Remember that he may enjoy playing peek-a-boo or looking for a hidden object. You can begin direct interaction with him by playing one of those games. Continue to involve his sister.

So far, you have 1) avoided separating him from his mother, and altered your body language to reduce his stranger anxiety; 2) familiarized him with you and your equipment by allowing him to play while you talked; 3) begun to make an ally of his mother and sister. As you procede with the exam you should 4) distract him using age appropriate play; 5) continue gradual familiarization with you, your equipment, and procedures; and 6) defer frightening, invasive, or painful parts of the exam until the end.

Throughout the chapters, examples of **preparation, observation,** and **modification** will be used. Experiment with various styles to see what works best for you.

INCORPORATING ASSESSMENT OF GROWTH AND DEVELOPMENT: BASIC PRINCIPLES

Student Tasks

1. Describe three methods to use in evaluating whether particular findings fall within or outside "the norm."
2. Define "following the curve" and "falling off the curve."

If you familiarize yourself with some basic principles of assessing growth and development, you will begin to acquire clinical "gestalt" with children. You ultimately want to answer the question: "Is this child normal?"

Every child progresses along each of the developmental continuums at his own unique rate. One child will gain weight quickly but be slow to speak. Another will acquire speech early but will be slow to walk. Sometimes progress is smooth; other times it proceeds in "fits and starts." How do you decide what is "normal" vs. "abnormal" for each particular child? Below are some principles to remember when examining children. They will help you begin to answer this question.

Compare a Child's Findings to Those of His Peers.

Many physical findings can be measured. Norms for these measurements have been established using data from large reference groups. To decide if a child's findings are "normal," you can compare his measurements to those of his peers. You can make these comparisons at **one point in time** (using cross-sectional data).

This kind of comparison is done at every well child visit. Height and weight are measured and "plotted" on the age- and sex-appropriate growth charts.

The growth charts (Figure 1.4) are for measurements from a *five-month-old male* who weighs *14½ lbs.* and measures *25¼ inches.* He is in the *25th* percentile for both length and weight. That is, when *compared to* a large group of normal American children, we expect that 75% of the population of five month old males will be longer and heavier than he, and 25% of that population will be lighter and shorter than he. That information tells you how he is doing at one point in time compared to his peers.

Norms have been established for many types of physical findings besides the ones mentioned above, e.g., head circumference, skin fold thickness, blood pressure, and even developmental milestones. The ones you will use most often are included in the Appendix.

Evaluate a Child's Rate of Progress over Time.

Measurable or observable findings such as body size, proportion, and even developmental abilities evolve along predictable continuums. Normal rates of progress along these continuums (established by large refer-

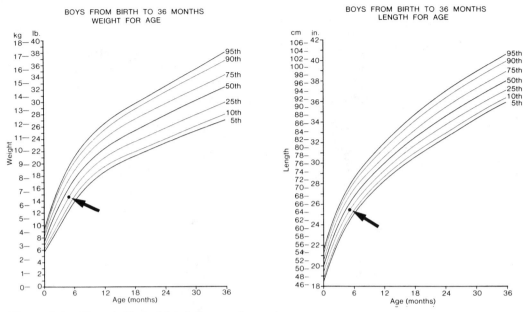

Figure 1.4.   Growth Charts Male infant age 5 months:
Weight 14.5 pounds = 25%
Length 25.25 inches = 25%
Used with permission from Hamill PVV, Drizd TA, Johnson CL, Reed RB, Roche AF, Moore WM.
Physical growth: National Center for Health Statistics percentiles. Am J Clin Nutr 1979;32:607–629.

ence populations) constitute what pediatricians call **"following the curve."** Each curve represents what constitutes normal progress for one segment of the population.

For example, Infant A is a five-month-old, 14½ lb., male infant who has been gaining steadily along the 25th percentile (Figure 1.5). He is evaluated as doing well. His weight is following a normal curve for infants in the 25th percentile. Infant B is a second five-month-old, 14½ lb., male. His weight is also at the 25th percentile. He would be evaluated as worrisome because he hasn't gained weight for the preceding two months (Figure 1.5). Even if you didn't know that infants should gain weight steadily during the first year, you would become alarmed when you plotted infant B's consecutive weights. You would see that he is no longer "following" his original percentile curve (the 75th percentile). This is known as **"falling off"** the curve and represents abnormal growth. You should also be aware that steady progress along any of the curves

within a normal range, whether along the 3rd or 95th percentile, is normal, and neither is "better" than the other.

Evaluate Specific Findings in a Child in the Context of the Rest of His Exam.

View deviations from expected in the context of the "whole child." One minor structural feature that departs from normal may have no significance if found in an otherwise healthy child. If, on the other hand, that child has several features that deviate from expected, then perhaps there is a syndrome which ties these findings together. (Syndromes are "recognizable patterns of structural and functional abnormalities or malformations that are known or presumed to be due to a single cause").[12] One example of a finding which may deviate from expected is an "upturned nose." (Now those of you out there with one, don't worry.)

As an isolated finding, an upturned nose may be familial or sporadic. In the presence of a broad forehead, flattened nasal bridge,

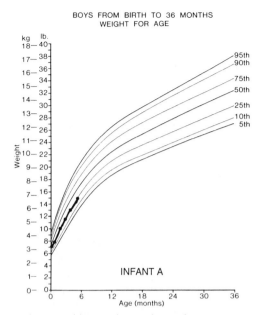

Figure 1.5A. Male age 5 months:
Weight is 14.5 pounds.
Weight is "following the curve."

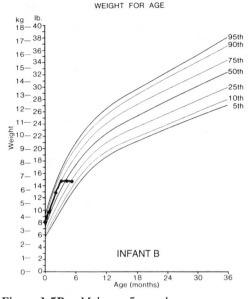

Figure 1.5B. Male age 5 months.
Weight is 14.5 pounds.
Weight is "falling off the curve."

Used with permission from Hamill PVV, Drizd TA, Johnson CL, Reed RB, Roche AF, Moore WM.
Physical growth: National center for Health Statistics percentiles. Am J Clin Nutr 1979;32:607–629.

epicanthal folds, elongated philtrum, and low-set ears, this may signal fetal hydantoin syndrome (maternal phenytoin ingestion during pregnancy) (Figure 1.6). I always like to use this example, because my daughter was born with a very upturned nose, clearly, not a "family" trait (Figure 1.6). I immediately worried! In her case, it was related to her in utero "Face" presentation against the cervix. Many of these variations of normal will be discussed, but the best way to learn after you have done your reading, is to examine as many children as possible.

THE "CONTENT" OF THE PEDIATRIC PHYSICAL EXAM

Student Task

1. List examples of physical examination data that may be obtained by observation.

You've just been introduced to the "style" of approaching children. You've also learned some things to think about while you're examining them. In the individual chapters both frameworks will be expanded upon, while reviewing the age-specific maneuvers of pediatric physical examinations.

The outline of the comprehensive physical exam is found, along with the comprehensive history, in the Appendix. Just as for the history, this is a suggested order for recording your findings, not for obtaining them. It also contains more information than you may need to obtain or record. The details are provided to help you decide that you haven't left out anything important.

Whatever order you choose, the physical exam always starts with a general assessment. The "tools" for this are your powers of observation. Remember that **observation** will give you as much information as laying hands on. Observation is helpful in guiding your history; it is helpful in guiding the "style" of interaction, but it is also most

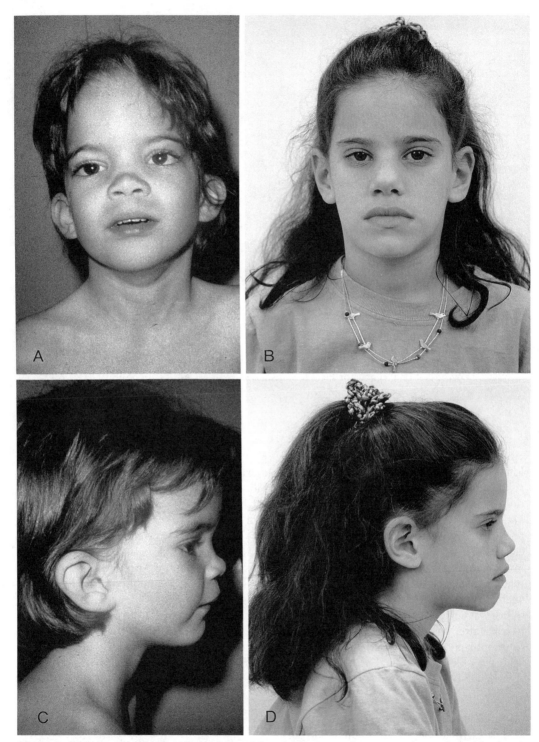

Figure 1.6A & C.   Fetal hydantoin syndrome. Note the presence of an upturned nose, broad forehead, flattened nasal bridge, epicanthal folds, elongated philtrum, and low-set ears. Photos 6A and 6C courtesy of Robert M. Greenstein, M.D.

Figure 1.6B & D.   Upturned nose as an isolated finding.

helpful in gathering "content" information about the physical examination. Observation begins the moment you encounter your patient and his family. For example, watching how smoothly a baby wakes and goes to sleep (called transitions of "state"), how well he makes eye contact, or how easily he is soothed, constitute important information that is gathered by observation. These observations would all be included in evaluations of development, family dynamics, or seriousness of an illness.

A final point, which is meant as a gentle, but very important, reminder: **Always begin your physical exam by washing your hands!**

Measurements on Pediatric Patients

Student Tasks

1. List the clinical circumstances in which each of the common pediatric measurements is utilized.
2. Describe the technique of obtaining each of the common pediatric measurements.

Measurements are one means of objective physical assessment. Below you will find explanations of the special techniques utilized in pediatrics to accomplish these assessments. Knowing how to measure children and how and what charts to plot these findings on allow you to begin interpreting how they are doing.

LENGTH/HEIGHT

Because of developmental stage (e.g., can't stand) and the uncooperative nature of young children, supine length is measured in children up to age two or three years. After that, standing height is used. If you are plotting **length** (measured in the supine position), use the charts that say: "**Birth to 36 months.**" If you are plotting **height** (measured in the erect position), use the charts that say: "**2 to 18 years.**" This is especially important to remember when you are measuring a toddler (as ages 2 to 3 can be plotted on either chart).

The infant is placed supine on a flat hard surface. The distance between the vertex (top of the head) and soles of the feet are measured. The best way to do this is to place either vertex or feet against a hard non-moveable board (that is at a 90° angle to the table surface). A second board at the other end of the child is moved towards the child with his legs extended until resistance is encountered. The distance between the two boards is the supine length. Two people are required to measure a squirming infant. This is an imprecise measurement in the full-term newborn and very young infant (first weeks of life). Term newborns are born with flexion contractures at the elbows, hips, and knees. Attempting to "stretch out" the legs in order to obtain an accurate length is an exercise in frustration for examiner and infant alike; it is usually unnecessary to force the issue with a healthy baby.

For standing height, have the child (shoes off) stand straight up with eyes looking straight ahead and feet together and the top of the head parallel to the floor. With a ruler flat across the top of the head, mark along the point that the ruler touches the scale or a place on the wall.

Plot length or height on the age- and sex-appropriate growth chart at the child's exact age. The diagonal lines on each chart give you the reference group percentiles.

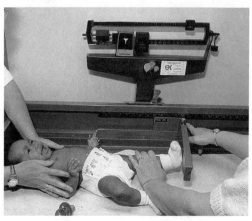

Figure 1.7. Measurement of supine length.

This should be done at each well child visit and may be done at other visits if there are concerns about growth or health.

Length and height charts are found in the Appendix.

WEIGHT

The infant is weighed (wearing a diaper) on a scale lying down. The older infant may sit up during this measurement. Children who are able to cooperate are weighed (in their underwear or gown) on a standard upright scale. Weight should be plotted on the age- and sex-appropriate charts.

Children are weighed at all well child visits. Weight is also measured in sick children, especially if their intake has been poor or when medication dosages need to be calculated.

Weight charts are found in the Appendix.

HEAD CIRCUMFERENCE

Head circumference is measured using a paper or cloth tape measure. Surround the head to obtain the maximal occipital-frontal circumference (OFC) (Figure 1.8). Younger children often have to be restrained for this procedure. You may need to repeat your measurements several times to make sure they are accurate. Plot your results on the sex-appropriate chart.

Head circumference is measured at every well child visit for the first year (the period of maximal brain growth), at every initial visit, or whenever there are concerns about growth or neurologic status.

Head circumference charts are found in the Appendix.

HEART RATE

Heart rate is determined either while listening directly over the precordium with a stethoscope or by palpating a convenient peripheral pulse. In an infant whose anterior fontanel is patent, you may also determine heart rate by counting the pulsations visible through the fontanel.

Normal heart rates decrease with advancing age throughout childhood. Normal heart rates encompass wide ranges. They also vary in an individual child with activity level, body temperature, illness, and stress.

Use the chart in the Appendix for reference.

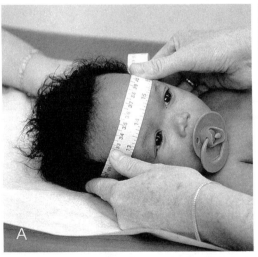 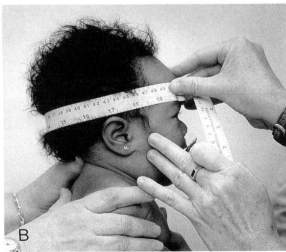

Figure 1.8A & B.   Measurement of head circumference. Anteriorly, the tape is positioned over the smooth area on the frontal bone just above the eyebrows. Posteriorly, it is positioned at the level of the occipital protuberance.

RESPIRATORY RATE

Respiratory rate is optimally determined with the child calm. This can be done either by auscultating the chest or observing the rise and fall of the chest (with the child unaware of what you are doing).

Respiratory rates (like heart rates) decrease with advancing age and encompass normal ranges. They, too, vary with activity level.

Use the chart in the Appendix for reference.

TEMPERATURE

Normal body temperature varies with age, activity, and time of day. Newborns have a slightly higher normal temperature than young children, who in turn have a slightly higher normal temperature than adolescents. The variation by age approximates 1° in total. More important is the diurnal variation in an individual child: body temperature rises to its highest level by early evening and falls to its lowest point at midnight. The average diurnal variation in temperature is usually at least one degree and may be as large as two or three degrees. Activity level, atmospheric temperature, and heavy clothing all influence body temperature in addition to illness. In the young infant, (under two months) subnormal temperature is sometimes a more ominous sign of illness than an elevated one.

Rectal temperatures are generally about a degree higher than oral. Forehead temperature strips are inaccurate. Axillary temperatures are said to be about 2° lower than rectal temperatures. Many pediatricians believe that axillary temperatures are inaccurate as well.

Rectal temperature is the best method to use until children are able to safely hold a mercury thermometer under their tongue. This will happen around age four or five. To obtain a rectal temperature, place the child prone in the parent's lap or on the examining table or bed. Insert approximately ¾ of an inch of the lubricated metal bulb end (this thermometer has the short bulb) into the rectum at an angle of approximately 25° to the floor, and hold it in place for one to two minutes. Holding the thermometer in place will be easier if the patient's buttocks are gently squeezed together.

Oral temperature is performed by asking the patient to place the long metal bulb under her tongue for two minutes.

Electronic thermometers are especially useful (they may be oral or rectal) (because they work faster) in the uncooperative patient. Some offices and hospitals have recently begun using a noninvasive device inserted into the ear canal which measures infrared energy emitted from the eardrum. At this time, the accuracy of this device in children is under investigation.[13]

Fahrenheit temperatures from approximately 97.5° to 100.4° rectal are generally considered in the normal range. Temperatures are taken routinely on newborns and hospitalized children. In the outpatient setting, they are generally reserved for children who are ill.

BLOOD PRESSURE

Blood pressure readings are performed at routine well child visits starting at the age of three. You may sometimes need to ascertain blood pressure readings on younger children if there are special concerns (e.g., heart or renal disease, a very ill infant, or if you have difficulty feeling the femoral pulse). A mercury-gravity sphygmomanometer is most commonly used in children beyond infancy, in the office, or inpatient setting (some facilities use Doppler ultrasonography or oscillometry). You may also use a portable aneroid manometer (many students do); just remember that this requires calibration against a mercury manometer once or twice a year.

Try to have the child as relaxed as possible (toddlers and older children should be seated). For routine measurement, use the

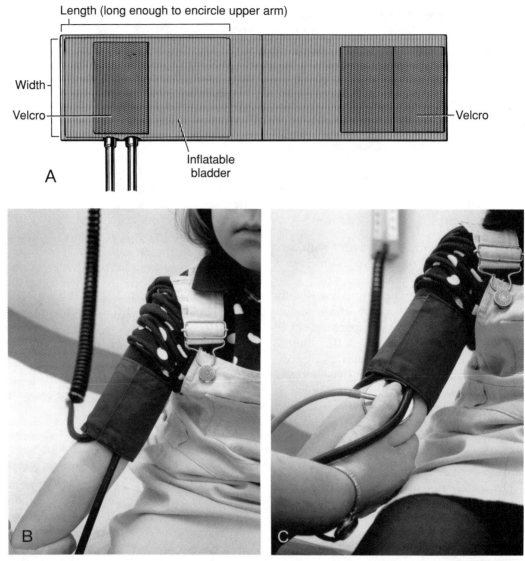

Figure 1.9. Determining the appropriate size and placement of the pediatric blood pressure cuff.
Figure 1.9A. The inner inflatable bladder should be long enough to completely encircle the upper arm.
Figure 1.9B & C. The cuff should be wide enough to cover approximately ¾ of the upper arm between the shoulder and the elbow allowing enough room to easily position the stethoscope at the antecubital fossa, and avoiding obstruction of the axilla.

right arm. Remind your patient that it will feel like a squeeze but that it won't hurt. You may also ask him to "help" you read the numbers by watching the mercury go up and then down.

The first rule of accurate blood pressure measurement is to insure that the proper cuff size is used. The cuff measurements refer to the inner inflatable bladder (not the outer cloth covering). The cuff (inflatable bladder) should completely encircle the circumference of the arm (with or without overlap). It should also be wide enough to cover about ¾ of the length of the upper arm. If you need to choose between two sizes, err on the larger size; it is virtually impossible to underestimate accurate blood pressure. Although thigh blood pressure measurements have not been extensively studied, the recommendations for cuff size selection in the thigh (using the popliteal artery) are the same as for the arm. Lower extremity systolic blood pressures (taken in the prone position) are normally higher (by approximately 10–30 mm.) than upper systolic extremity blood pressures.

Position your stethoscope lightly over the brachial artery (the lower border of the cuff should begin above the antecubital fossa). Inflate the cuff 20–30 mm. above the point at which the radial pulse disappears. As you begin to deflate the cuff, the point of onset (K1) of tapping sounds (Korotkoff sounds) corresponds to the systolic blood pressure. With further deflation, the onset (K4) of low-pitched muffled sounds occurs, and, finally, the disappearance of sounds (K5) is reached. Both K4 and K5 have been used as the diastolic pressure points. In children, K5 is sometimes difficult to obtain (it is easier to distinguish in adolescents). Therefore, K4 diastolic BPs are used in the standards for infants and children up to age 12, and K5 diastolic BPs are used in the standards for adolescents 13–18 years of age.[14]

Like other measurements in children, blood pressures change with age. There is a gradual progression upwards with advancing age. Blood pressures also rise with anxiety.

Normal values are found in the Appendix.

BEFORE YOU CONTINUE

Before you continue, take a moment to reflect on what you have accomplished thus far. From this point on, as you approach the nursery or ward, you will be less distracted by the physical environment and therefore better equipped to concentrate on the tasks at hand. By familiarizing yourself with the goals and mechanics of pediatric clinical encounters, you have acquired the "blueprint" from which to proceed. The specifics, or age-related content will be much easier to grasp and recall, now that you are prepared!

References

1. Solomon, R. Pediatric experiences in year II clinical sciences. E. Lansing, Michigan: Department of Pediatrics and Human Development, College of Human Medicine, Michigan State University, 1986.
2. Thompson HC. Can pediatrics meet the challenge of social ill health? Am J Dis Child 1987;141:884.
3. Forman MA, Hetznecker WH, Dunn JM. Assessment and interviewing. In: Vaughan VC, McKay RJ, Behrman RE, eds. Nelson textbook of pediatrics. 11th ed. Philadelphia: W.B. Saunders, 1979:80–83.
4. Dower JC. The pediatric interview. In: Rudolph AM, ed. Pediatrics. 17th ed. Norwalk, Connecticut: Appleton-Century-Crofts, 1982:19–20.
5. Telzrow RW. Anticipatory guidance in pediatric practice. J Cont Educ Pediatr 1978;20:14–27.
6. Ginsburg H, Oppers S. Piaget's theory of intellectual development: an introduction. Englewood Cliffs, NJ: Prentice Hall, Inc., 1969.
7. Chess S, Hassibi M. Theory of cognitive development of Jean Piaget. In: Rudolph AM, ed. Pediatrics. 17th ed. Norwalk, Connecticut: Appleton-Century-Crofts, 1982:48–49.
8. Moss JR. Helping young children cope with the physical examination. Pediatr Nurs 1981;March/April:17–20.
9. Galazka SS. Clinical magic and the art of examining children. J Fam Pract 1984;18:229–232.
10. Apley J. Listening and talking to patients. Br Med J 1980;281:1116–1117.
11. Smilkstein G. The pediatric lap examination. J Fam Pract 1977;4:743–745.
12. Saal HM, Cassidy SB. Genetic disorders and birth defects. In: Dworkin PH, ed. The national medical series for independent study: pediatrics. New York: John Wiley & Sons, Inc., 1987:138.
13. Rhoads FA, Grandner J. Assessment of an aural infrared sensor for body temperature measurement in children. Clin Pediatr 1990;29:112–115.
14. Task Force on Blood Pressure Control in Children: Report of the second task force on blood pressure control in children—1987. Pediatrics 1987;79:1–4.

Most of the concepts discussed in this chapter are in the common genre of pediatricians. General references for further reading are provided in the appendix.

CHAPTER 2

Newborn

THE PHYSICAL EXAM OF THE NEWBORN
Student Task

1. Examine a healthy newborn.

After you've reviewed the available nursery data (we'll fill in the details later), familiarized yourself with the set-up, and have "scrubbed," walk over to your newborn's bedside.

Wait! Don't touch her quite yet! Just look at her for a minute. She will spend much of the first twenty-four hours sleeping. After that, she will begin to wake in a cyclical pattern for feeds. Even in a brand new newborn we can observe differences in temperament. As you proceed through your exam, note how easily (or suddenly) she makes transitions from waking to sleeping, or fussing to calming (use your powers of **observation** for this **general assessment**). Some infants do this handily and calmly, while others react suddenly and uneasily. These transitions from "state" to "state" begin to give you a feel for differences in newborn behavioral styles. You will also learn (as do new parents) that, in some babies, these patterns of behavior change from day to day or hour by hour, while others are quite stable from the very beginning. The most predictable thing about newborns is their unpredictability.

I know you are anxious to get started (and perhaps anxious is the right word), but hold off for another minute. Right now you may feel very intimidated. As you look around, it seems that everyone else knows more than you do. The nurses handle babies "properly" without a second thought. Your resident or instructor will want you to make "observations" about "your" baby, when you are more concerned about how you are going to pick her up and turn her over the first time! Please remember:

1. We all (and I mean all) had to be taught how to handle a newborn at one time! By gently cradling the back of the head with one hand and the body with the other, you won't get into trouble (you'll be amazed at how much easier it will feel the second time). (See Fig. 2.1 on p. 23.)
2. "Your" baby is going to cry from being disturbed at some point in your exam. That is a predictable and normal reaction of the newborn to being disturbed.
3. You won't break the baby by touching her.
4. You are equipped with a lot of substantive information! You've just spent years acquiring that information. Be assured you will soon be able to use some of that information.

O.K., now that we've identified your normal state, let's go back to that of the newborn . . .

Is she quiet? If so, you can listen to her breathing and count her respirations per minute. The usual rate is approximately 40 times per minute (range approximately 30–75); it slows during quiet sleep and may go much higher if she is agitated or sick. Short pauses are normal. Can you hear any noises other than quiet breathing? If you do, she may have an anomaly (an abnormal structural feature) along her respiratory tree (e.g., in her trachea or nose).[1]

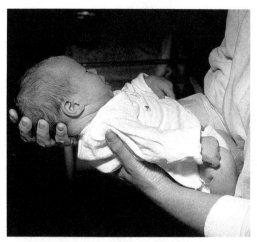

Figure 2.1. Cradle the newborn's head in one hand and support the body with the other hand.

The baby will be swaddled and lying on her side or abdomen. If you give into the temptation to turn her onto her back and undress her, you will awaken her. She'll probably cry. Hold off. While she's still sleeping, sneak into the part of the exam that most requires her quiet cooperation.

Cardiorespiratory

In the newborn exam, this is the major deviation from a "head to toe" order. Gently open the blanket and lift up the shirt just enough to "sneak" your warmed stethoscope onto the chest. Listen to the heart. This deviates from the usual order of the cardiac exam in which you would inspect and palpate the precordium first. Make sure the heart is loudest in the left chest (otherwise, the heart may be situated on the right!) Listen all over the precordium, and to the right side of the chest, and then in the back, too. Evaluate the rate for beats per minute and regularity. The usual heart rate is 120 beats per minute (approximate range 90–160). It will be on the lower end of the range if the child is sleeping. As in older children, you may find the rate varies with respiration. This is called sinus arrhythmia. (The heart rate speeds up during inspiration and slows with expiration). Actually, this is rarely found in newborns (but may be). Remember it when you examine older infants and children.

Listen to the first (S1) and second (S2) sounds. Even though the rate is quite a bit faster than in adults, with practice you will find it possible to evaluate each of these sounds as distinct entities. In the newborn, S1 is usually a single sound. S2 splits during inspiration (this reflects the normal nonsimultaneous closure of, first, the aortic and then the pulmonic valves). With a fast heart rate, this is very difficult to evaluate and takes a lot of practice. This will be easier to distinguish in older children because their heart rates are slower.

Once you have identified the two heart sounds, listen for murmurs, extra sounds, or clicks, using both the bell and the diaphragm. It is not uncommon to hear an innocent murmur in the first 24 to 48 hours of life.

An **innocent murmur,** by definition, is a murmur that is associated with no underlying cardiac disease. There are several innocent murmurs to listen for in each age group. Except for the venous hum (to be described later in the young child), an innocent murmur is never heard in diastole and is never associated with other adventitious cardiac sounds (e.g., clicks or rubs) or other signs of cardiac disease (e.g., cyanosis, absent pulses, etc.).

The etiologies of most innocent murmurs heard in the neonate are uncertain but are thought to be related to either blood flow turbulance produced by a closing ductus arteriosus or from falling pulmonary vascular resistance. These are soft (usually not louder than grade 2/6), blowing, and occupy the ejection period of systole (beginning after S1); most are heard best along the upper left sternal border. Most of these murmurs disappear within a few days.

The murmur of **peripheral pulmonic stenosis** (PPS) is the most easily diagnosed specific innocent neonatal murmur. It is a short, midsystolic blowing murmur (not louder than grade 2/6), and is best heard along the distribution of the peripheral pulmonary arteries. Thus it may be heard in the front of the chest, the axillae, and back. The key to identifying this murmur is that if it is heard in the right chest as clearly as in the left, then you can be fairly certain that it originates (not radiates to) from the right chest as well as the left. Confirmation that this is an innocent murmur is confirmed when the murmur disappears; this occurs by approximately age 3 months.

This baby is probably waking up by now. By continuing to be very gentle, try to complete your cardiorespiratory exam. Offer her a pacifier to keep her calm. Palpate for heaves, lifts or thrills, and the PMI (point of maximal impulse) which should be at the 4th left intercostal space, just left of the midclavicular line.

If you haven't already done so, count the respiratory rate. Newborns have normal pauses in their breathing cycles, but these should not exceed 20 seconds per pause nor should they be accompanied by bradycardia. Pauses that exceed 20 seconds and pauses of any length when accompanied by limpness, pallor, cyanosis, or bradycardia and requiring vigorous stimulation, are defined as apnea of infancy.[2]

Listen for the normally clear or bronchovesicular breath sounds. (The brand new newborn, who is just a few hours old might have some scattered crackles. These disappear within hours.) By now, you've bothered her enough to evoke a cry. It should sound strong and lusty.

❷ A term baby sounds hoarse when she cries, but has no other symptoms of respiratory distress. In your review of the records, you noted that there was "meconium" passed prior to delivery. (Meconium passage prior to delivery is a sign of fetal distress). Why is she hoarse? If you haven't spent time in the delivery room (DR) yet, this isn't really a fair question. The reason is that she was laryngoscoped in the DR to check for aspiration of meconium below the level of the vocal cords. This procedure may produce transient laryngeal inflammation and mild hoarseness and/or stridor. In newborns, stridor sounds like a high-pitched crowing. The hoarseness and stridor will resolve in a few days. If there was no history of this procedure, (and there is hoarseness with or without stridor), then you must think of an anomaly of or around the larynx (i.e., congenital subglottic stenosis, in which the subglottic airway may be narrowed, or a vascular ring, by pressing onto the airway might do this, too. A paralysed vocal cord is another more common cause for hoarseness.)

You may also hear some nasal sounds. Mild nasal congestion, with residual amniotic fluid is common in healthy newborns. Babies resolve this very mild stuffiness by sneezing. Marked nasal congestion is seen in babies with congenital syphilis beginning at the end of the first week of life, and very frequent sneezing is seen in infants with narcotic withdrawal. Most babies breathe through their noses (vs. mouths) during the early months of life. If the nasal passages are blocked (i.e., choanal atresia is a congenital bony or membranous obstruction of the posterior nasal airway), the baby is forced to attempt to breath though the mouth. When the mouth is closed (e.g., when occluded by a nipple during feeds) the baby with bilateral choanal atresia will display severe respiratory distress, usually with apnea and cyanosis. To rule-out choanal atresia which may be unilateral and sometimes asymptomatic in the newborn period, we pass a flexible catheter through each side of the nose soon after birth.

You should not hear diffuse crackles or wheezes. Respiratory distress in the newborn may result from intrinsic pulmonary disease (i.e., respiratory distress syndrome of the premature infant, pneumothorax, or pneumonia), cardiac disease (e.g., congestive heart failure), or from a more systemic process (e.g., sepsis). Babies with **respiratory distress breathe very quickly** (or have too **lengthy pauses**, i.e., apnea), and often **grunt** on expiration (I don't have to tell you what that sounds like . . . it sounds like a grunt!) and may have **intercostal, sub-costal, or supraclavicular retractions.** The adventitious sounds you hear on auscultation will depend on the etiology of the respiratory distress (e.g., possible crackles in pneumonia; with sepsis you may not hear any adventitious sounds). Babies in distress may also have **nasal flaring** (widening of the alae on inspiration). As pulmonary failure worsens, you may observe **cyanosis of mucous membranes.** In other words, they "work" to breathe, and it is usually fairly obvious beyond the rapid respiratory rate stage.

Roll the baby onto one side or another and auscultate in the back. When you are finished listening, roll the baby on to her back.

While you're still thinking about the cardiorespiratory exam, feel the upper extremity pulses and femoral pulses. Simultaneously palpate both brachial arteries for equal volume and timing; then palpate the right brachial and femoral arteries. A healthy newborn has strong (but not bounding) pulses. A child with decreased cardiac output will have poor pulses. The femoral pulses are palpable at the inguinal line or just below (on the very upper medial thigh). In a squirming infant who has a degree of normal hip flexion contracture, finding the femoral pulse isn't always possible. If you encounter difficulty with this, feel for the dorsalis pedis pulse. If the femorals are very weak or absent, or delayed when compared simultaneously to the right brachial pulse, (and you cannot find a dorsalis pedis pulse either), suspect an obstruction in the aorta (i.e., **coarctation**). If there is concern about the cardiovascular exam or general appearance of the baby, ask for assistance in taking your baby's blood pressure. The skin, mucous membranes, and liver/spleen exams also have components that are pertinent to the cardio-vascular exam. We'll review these shortly.

Now you are ready to go back to the head and examine the rest from head to toe. In this age group, you don't have to reason with or cajole your patient. Just choose an order that's easy to remember (e.g., cardio-respiratory followed by head to toe). Some pediatricians also palpate the abdomen before they return to the head. In addition, you will probably choose to defer the hip examination to the very end of the exam (most babies cry with this exam).

The newborn exam is really a screen for congenital anomalies. A congenital anomaly is an abnormal structural feature that is present (but not necessarily apparent) at birth.[1] Congenital anomalies may result from the influence of: abnormal genes, teratogens (e.g., drugs taken by the mother), abnormal intrauterine forces (e.g., fibroid tumors), and events occurring during pregnancy (e.g., infection, vascular accidents, etc.). We will be discussing many examples of these as we proceed through the newborn exam. In the introductory chapter we spoke about evaluating findings within the context of the "whole child." Findings must also be evaluated within the context of the patient's family. What may seem like an unusual facial finding (e.g., a funny shaped nose, or a dimple in an unusual location), may in fact be a family trait. This is often reassuring. Just be careful not to gain too much of a sense of false security. **Some family traits are merely minor cosmetic issues. Some family traits are important congenital anomalies** which have underlying and possibly significant associated problems. In either case, remember to look at mom, dad, and sibs, too.

Hair

Does she have a lot or a little hair? Note also the color, texture, and distribution of hair. Lanugo, the fine downy hair which covers the fetus, progressively diminishes as the infant approaches term. Aside from lanugo, the variation in hair quality and quantity varies enormously from baby to baby. In normal infants some of this variation is familial. If your baby has no hair, check to see if she has eyebrows. If these are absent too, and this isn't an extremely premature baby, you may be seeing evidence of a birth defect. (The **ectodermal dysplasias** are a group of inherited disorders involving abnormalities of hair, skin derivatives, and other ectodermally derived structures). Other rare disorders are associated with abnormalities in color or texture of hair. Still other disorders are associated with abnormal patterns of hair. For example, more than one hair whorl is considered a dysmorphic feature. In the presence of multiple hair whorls, other craniofacial anomalies should be carefully searched for.

Head

Many newborns have "battle scars" from intrauterine life, labor, or delivery. These are much more common than anomalies. Many of these fade rather quickly but can be alarming and sometimes disappointing to new parents. Our job is to recognize these and reassure when it is appropriate to do so.

A common site for battle scars are the head and face. Inspect and feel the head all around. A good approach for the head (for the rest of the exam too), is to **compare sides** (right and left). Note any asymmetries or bulges. Common causes of irregularities are:

MOLDING

The head will look or feel slightly asymmetric or elongated. This is from pressure on the presenting part (more common after vaginal deliveries).

CAPUT

This is edema of the scalp tissues (also from pressure). The swelling crosses the midline and is usually found on the top or back of the head. It will feel somewhat firm, but ill-defined in circumference, and will pit with pressure applied by your fingertip.

CEPHALOHEMATOMA

This is a subperiosteal hematoma. This type of swelling does not cross the midline (limited by suture lines). It will feel firm and more circumscribed than a caput. The center

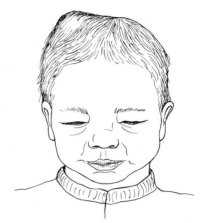

Figure 2.2.   Cephalohematoma.

of the swelling may have a "mushy" or tense consistency depending on the amount of blood contained within it. A cephalohematoma may be associated with a linear skull fracture; this is usually clinically inapparent. (The clinician should palpate for a depression in the skull contour which may indicate the less common, but more serious, association of a depressed skull fracture.)

These battle scars gradually resolve over days to weeks. The cephalohematoma may leave behind small, hard (calcium-containing) nodules of no significance.

The key to the "benign" swellings is to distinguish them from more important swellings: **encephaloceles** and **meningoceles**. Make sure that there is bone underneath the "usual swellings." That tells you that there is probably no brain communication with the scalp (as with an encephalocele).

❓ **A term newborn (Figure 2.3) delivered a few hours ago has a huge cone-shaped swelling on the top of his head that crosses the midline. It pits and has skull underneath it. The mom is appalled and worries that her child will look like a Martian. (You are fairly worried, too.) The baby is otherwise well. What will you tell her? . . . That's right . . . because you have read the delivery sheet, you have found out that this baby was delivered via "vacuum" extraction. The swelling is a huge caput. Tell her that this is**

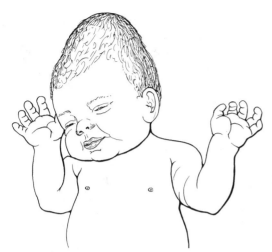

Figure 2.3. Quiz: Newborn with cone-shaped swelling.

common after this type of delivery and that it will resolve.

Run your fingers along the suture lines and the fontanelles. (Figure 2.4) Cranial sutures are not fused at birth. Fusion occurs many years after cranial bones have stopped growing. Molding may push cranial bones together so that they feel fused or even overlapping. Note the feeling along the suture lines. Very marked overriding (ridging) of sutures or marked bony asymmetries of the cranium are abnormal. Ridging when

secondary to molding and not to an underlying abnormality like premature fusion of the sutures, will resolve during a period of weeks to several months. The pediatrician will follow this with periodic exams to be sure that this occurs. The opposite finding, extremely wide separation of sutures (more than a finger tip), may mean there is increased intracranial pressure (as you might see in hydrocephalus), especially if the head circumference is abnormally large.

Don't be afraid to outline the sizes of the anterior and posterior fontanelles with your fingers. With practice you will be able to estimate their size. The anterior (or diamond-shaped) one is about 2 × 2 cm. (maybe 3 × 4 cm.), and the posterior fontanelle is usually about a fingertip open. Abnormally large fontanelles may be seen with hydrocephalus (and some skeletal, chromosomal, congenital, and metabolic disorders); small fontanelles may be seen in such conditions as microcephaly and hyperparathyroidism. Small and large fontanelles may also be normal variants.

There shouldn't be any bulging visible or palpable through the fontanelles. Check for true fontanelle bulging only when the baby is held upright (to eliminate the effects of gravity) and is not crying or struggling. True bulging of the fontanelles may be a sign of increased intracranial pressure.

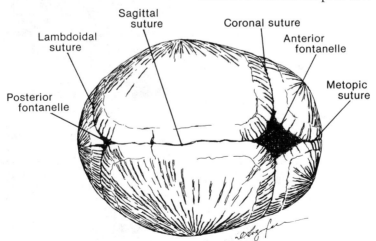

Figure 2.4. Cranial sutures and fontanelles. Reproduced with permission. Willms JL, Lewis J, eds. Introduction to clinical medicine. Baltimore: Williams & Wilkins, 1991:138.

Measure the head circumference using the paper tape measure.

❓ How do you measure head circumference? . . . Obtain the maximal circumference by surrounding the head with the tape at the levels of the forehead and occipital prominence (where the skull bulges out a little).

After you have estimated by baby's gestational age (I will teach you to do this a little later on), plot the head circumference measurement on the head circumference graph. Microcephaly is defined as a head circumference that is more than 2 standard deviations below the norm for age. A small head reflects a small brain. Macrocephaly is a large head circumference, or a head which measures more than 2 standard deviations above the norm for age. A large head may be a normal/familial variant. It may also result from hydrocephalus. A macrocephalic head may have a small, normal, or large brain inside.

You may also find a small healing scab on the scalp. This is from the site of insertion of the fetal monitor used to monitor baby's heart rate during labor. It will heal over a week's time.

Face

Next examine the baby's face. Think about your **general assessment.** Is there anything unusual about the appearance? Does the baby appear: placid, alert, angry? There may be linear purplish bruises. These are forceps marks and are also not permanent. Depending on the age of the infant and on the innate coloring, the skin may be pink, reddish, or pale-appearing. Pallor may be real or merely reflect "fair" skin tone. Pallor is especially difficult to assess in infants whose natural skin coloring is dark. To confirm or rule out pallor, it is helpful to check the palpebral conjunctivae (by everting the lower lids). The blood vessels should have a strong pink color. If these too are pale, the infant may be truly anemic. Pallor may also reflect impend-

ing shock, but in an otherwise well appearing baby, this is unlikely.

There may be clusters of small yellow-whitish papules on the skin, mostly on the bridge of the nose, chin or cheeks (Figure 2.5). These papules, which result from retained keratin and sebum, are called **milia** and are transient. Note facial jaundice (you may need to use natural sunlight to decide). Jaundice in the neonate generally becomes obvious on the face first. As the bilirubin rises, jaundice "spreads" caudally to include the rest of the body and also the sclerae.

Look at the eyes, ears, nose, and mouth, always first looking for symmetry.

Ears

Ears are examined for their placement, shape, size, and patency. You certainly know where the general location should be. If they are normally "set," when you draw an imaginary horizontal line through the medial canthi (inner corner of the eyes) across to the ears, at least one tenth to one fifth of the total ear height will fall above the line. If less than that amount, and definitely if the entire ear falls below the line, the ears are said to be **"low-set"**. This determination can be made in patients of all ages (Figure 2.6).

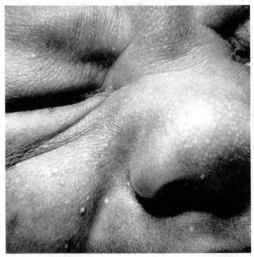

Figure 2.5. Milia. Photo courtesy of Douglas H. MacGilpin, M.D.

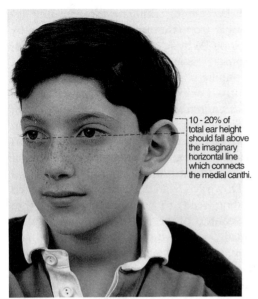

10 - 20% of total ear height should fall above the imaginary horizontal line which connects the medial canthi.

Figure 2.6. Determining whether or not the ears are low-set.

This observation is important, because low set ears are associated with renal and auditory abnormalities and some syndromes. Total height of the ear may also be important. If in doubt about whether an ear is too small, consult a genetics text for the standards. **Now that you know how to determine whether or not an ear is "low-set," go back to the photos of the child with fetal hydantoin syndrome in Chapter 1 (Figure 1.6) and practice the method I just described.**

The ear should also be placed in a vertical plane relative to the head. If the top of the helix appears posteriorly rotated or if there are missing contours, this too could signal one of the aforementioned problems. The normal curves of the ear have been described for you on adults. If the helix is very pliable (feeling as if it lacks cartilage), the baby may be premature (more about that when you learn to estimate gestational age). Note any pits or tags. These are found anywhere on the body but are most common on or near the ears. Occasionally, these will be associated with branchial cleft abnormalities (but are also found in normal children). Finally,

make sure that the ear canal appears patent. During the first few days of life, the canal will contain some amniotic fluid. It is usually unnecessary to use the otoscope for healthy newborns.

Eyes

The eyelids may be very swollen and have an underlying mucoid or slightly yellowish discharge. This reaction, which is a chemical conjunctivitis, is often seen in the first 24 to 48 hours of life after instillation of silver nitrate drops. The drops are instilled at birth to prevent gonoccocal conjunctivitis. There are also infectious causes for swelling and drainage, but these usually begin later during the first week of life.

The baby may open her eyes spontaneously for you. If so, or even if not, say "hi." Even at this age, some newborns respond by opening their eyes and/or turning their heads to the sound of the human voice. This is one of the pleasures experienced by new parents. The newborn very quickly learns to discriminate the sounds of her own mother's voice. As baby, mom and dad begin the attachment process known as "bonding," this preferential reaction intensifies.

If you lift her upright (support her axillae in the crook of your hands while cradling the back of her head with your fingertips), she should reflexively open her eyes (Figure 2.7). While she's upright, move her from side to side and up and down; finally, tip her head and upper body backwards (continue to cradle her head in your hands), then return her to the upright position. During these maneuvers, observe that her eyes move in all directions. You will also observe that her eyes will deviate in the direction opposite to the direction her head is moving (doll's eye reflex).

Note the shape, symmetry, and size of her eyes. Check the lids for ptosis. There are many references for measurements of the eyes (as for the ears). One of the most important is the **interpupillary distance.** This helps you to decide if the eyes are too close together (**hypotelorism**) or if they are too far apart (**hypertelorism**). Another is the distance from the medial canthus (you learned this term earlier) to the lateral canthus of each eye. This is known as the **palpebral fissure width.** This helps you to decide if the eye openings are wide enough. Look up the exact normal values for interpupillary distance and palpebral fissure width in a reference text, if the eyes look unusual to you. In practice, with normal babies, we evaluate these just by looking at the baby. If you force yourself to make these types of observations on all patients, you will eventu-

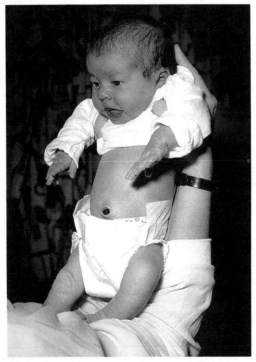

Figure 2.7. When the infant is held upright she reflexively opens her eyes.

ally learn to discriminate the probably abnormal from the probably normal just by looking. Why is this important? Many syndromes are associated with abnormal interpupillary distances or palpebral fissure widths. For example, short palpebral fissures are seen in fetal alcohol syndrome.

Sometimes there is a little fold of skin covering the medial canthus (called an **epicanthal fold**). This has significance only if associated with other abnormal findings (as in Down syndrome). Remember, an isolated finding needs to be thought about within the context of the "whole" child and family. Finally, while you are drawing imaginary lines, try another one though the medial and lateral canthus of each eye. This line determines the **slant of the palpebral fissure.** If this line slants upwards as it moves from medial to lateral, then the palpebral fissure has a mongoloid slant (or if it slants downward as it moves laterally this is called an antimongoloid slant) (Figure 2.8). A mongoloid or antimongoloid slant may be related to the patient's family or racial origin, it may be an isolated finding, or it may be part of a syndrome. For example, patients with Down syndrome have palpebral fissures with mongoloid slants. Patients with Treacher Collins syndrome may have antimongoloid slants (Figure 2.8).

Look at the globes. Are they both present? (Believe it or not, this has been missed.) Do they appear to bulge? Are they the same size? Are the irises present? Are they complete? Look for gaps (or colobomas) in each structure of the eyes. Are the pupils present and equal in size? The newborn pupillary

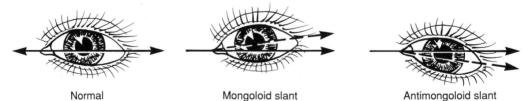

Normal   Mongoloid slant   Antimongoloid slant

Figure 2.8. Determining the angle of the palpebral fissure. Reproduced with permission. DeMeyer W. Technique of the neurologic examination: a programmed text. 3rd ed. New York: McGraw Hill, 1980:3.

response to light may be very sluggish, but it is present. Even very young newborns can see shadows and shapes, particularly at a distance of about 12 inches. If you have a very alert, calm infant, you may want to see if she will fix and follow. She should be able to fix on your face and follow it up to 90° in either direction from the midline. While holding her upright, pay attention to whether or not she fixes on your face; then while holding her steady, move your head horizontally from side to side (and vertically up and down), and watch to see if her eyes follow your movements. If you aren't successful, try it again. If she appears to look away from you, then she isn't fixing. Don't use a flashlight for this, as she will probably blink in response, then shut her eyes tightly until you move the bright light away from her.

Check for a red reflex bilaterally; you probably won't be able to see much other funduscopic detail. At minimum, assess the equality of color and clarity of the red reflex. The corneas should not be cloudy (as in congenital glaucoma or with a cataract). If the cornea isn't cloudy and you can see the red reflex clearly, then there are probably no cataracts. This is important, because some cataracts should be removed very early in life in order for normal sight to develop. Congenital cataracts are seen in a variety of conditions such as congenital infections (i.e., congenital rubella).

Examine the sclerae and conjunctivae. The sclerae may be dotted with focal hemorrhages. These too are "battle scars" and resolve without treatment. The sclerae should otherwise be white or blueish white. Note scleral icterus (we talked about this earlier). Very blue sclerae, which don't become white (as a child grows older), are associated with a spectrum of syndromes of "brittle bones" and deafness called **osteogenesis imperfecta.** These children may be born with fracture deformities. An otherwise normal child with intensely blue sclerae will be followed by her pediatrician for the possible appearance of these problems later on.

❓ In addition to the uncommon presentation of findings associated with osteogenesis imperfecta, what other physical findings would make you wonder about "your" baby's hearing? . . . That's it! A malformed or misplaced ear . . . Too obvious? Good! Then you are acquiring the "eye" of a pediatrician!

Back to the baby's eyes. If you have lifted her up and put her through her paces you've watched her eyes move in all directions. There is usually a tendency towards periodic misalignment of the eyes in the newborn period. The eyes will cross periodically. This crossing should disappear by approximately age three months. As a result of this early phenomenon, most types of strabismus, or abnormal ocular alignment, will not be diagnosed by the pediatrician during the newborn period. Strabismus, which involves fixed paralysis of an extraocular muscle (not the most common form of strabismus), may be diagnosed in a newborn if a careful examiner has attempted to observe the eyes move in all directions of gaze. There will be a fixed limitation of extraocular movement in one or more direction, depending on which muscles are involved.

Nose

Make sure both nares appear patent. As mentioned earlier, some sneezing (the way newborns blow their noses) is common. Feel for an intact nasal bridge and bone. It should appear midline, although sometimes there can be swelling and mild asymmetry from the birth battle. Some otolaryngologists prefer to repair marked septal deviations in the newborn period. Noses, too, may be a signal to other abnormalities (e.g., a markedly beaked nose is seen in **Seckels syndrome;** a very upturned nose can be seen in idiopathic hypercalcemia of infancy). Just remember these findings do not occur in isolation. They merely signal you to look more closely at the rest.

The distance between the nares and the top of the lip (the **philtrum**) has also been standardized. If it appears unusually short or elongated, measure it. Elongated philtrums are seen in **fetal alcohol syndrome.**

Mouth

By now she's probably crying again. Make sure you watch her mouth when she's crying. If only one side turns down, this may mean she has an absence of the depressor anguli oris muscle, a defect that is part of the **asymmetric crying facies** syndrome which has associated cardiac and other defects. Interestingly, the abnormal paralyzed side is the side that does not turn down. If you notice an asymmetry, make sure the rest of the face is symmetric. Otherwise, you might miss another problem, a facial nerve palsy, which will also manifest as palpebral fissure asymmetry (wider fissure on the paralyzed side) and a flattening of the naso-labial fold (with the face deviating to the nonparalyzed side). This may occur from damage to the facial nerve during a forceps delivery. (Look in front of the ear for the purple staining of forceps bruising).

The lips and tongue should also be inspected for adequacy of size and for presence of "pits." You guessed it, more syndrome association. The lips and tongue should be pink. Sometimes the skin surrounding the lips (called the perioral skin) may be slightly cyanotic. This **perioral cyanosis** is usually **normal** and is associated with the newborn's peripheral vascular instability. If the lips and tongue are blue or purple, then this represents true cyanosis (arterial oxygen desaturation) and requires medical attention.

Feel the entire length of the palate in addition to looking at it. In some nurseries, especially where the incidence of AIDS is high, you may be required to wear a glove for this part of the exam. Inspect the uvula, pharynx, and gingivae. Your flashlight and tongueblade will be helpful here. A cleft of the lip or hard palate will be obvious. A cleft of the soft palate will not necessarily be. A submucous cleft of the soft palate or a bifid (split) uvula may be associated with speech and hearing difficulties. As you feel the palate, feel for the normal midline ridge of the hard palate. It should not have a very high concavity (or arch); this too is seen in association with certain congenital syndromes. There may be some whitish papules near the junction of the hard and soft palates or on the gum lines. The papules on the palate (located on either side of the median raphe) are known as **Epstein's pearls.** The papules on the gum lines (inclusion cysts) are called **epithelial pearls.** Both types of "pearls" are shed spontaneously within weeks to months; neither have clinical significance. Other soft tissue tumors in the newborn mouth (i.e., an epulis or a tumor originating from the gums) may need to be excised because they grow larger and aren't spontaneously shed. Occasionally, a tooth will have erupted (called, as expected, a natal tooth). This requires an x-ray to determine if this is a deciduous tooth, or just an "extra" (supernumerary tooth). If it is loose, it will have to be pulled, because of the risk of aspiration to the neonate. Consultation with a dentist, preferably a pediatric dentist, in this circumstance is important.

The tongue should fit easily inside the mouth. If it doesn't, then either (now don't be insulted by this next statement) the tongue is too big (i.e., **Beckwith syndrome**), or the jaw is too small (i.e., **Pierre Robin syndrome**). Either of these problems can interfere with breathing and feeding. Finally, it may appear that the tongue does not reach out of the mouth very far because of a tight or shortened frenulum. In the old days, we called this "tongue tied" and in our infinite wisdom we cut the frenulum (believe it or not, with a scissors) before the baby was discharged from the nursery. Fortunately, we've learned to reserve our limited surgical attempts in this area. A tight frenulum rarely produces problems for speaking or eating. In the vast majority of cases the tongue grows and the frenulum stretches out without any interference from us. In the rare circumstances of interference with normal speech development, a surgical procedure will be considered during late childhood.

Let her suck on your finger (**sucking reflex**). She should be able to make a nice seal, and exert some firm pressure. Now stroke the skin just lateral to the side of the mouth in a direction towards the cheek. If she is calm, she will turn her head towards the side that you have stroked and begin to suck. This is called the **rooting reflex.** Finally, you may notice that her jaw quivers for short periods. In the newborn, this is normal.

Neck, Thorax, and Upper Extremities

Now it is time to remove the tee shirt and take a good **look,** and **feel** of the neck, clavicles, upper extremities, and chest. There should be no bulges from the neck (as you would see if cysts or hemangiomas were present). The newborn's thyroid isn't visible unless it is enlarged. A midline neck mass may be a goiter or, more commonly, a thyroglossal duct cyst. (The only way to pick up a subtle goiter is to hyperextend the baby's neck). Make sure that there is some neck visible. Girls with **Turner syndrome** (a chromosomal disorder in females in which there is only 1 X or one normal X chromosome) the neck may be webbed. There may be a few palpable cervical lymph nodes (and perhaps femoral ones, too). These should feel pea-sized, soft, and mobile.

The newborn neck is quite supple. There should be no limitation to passive motion in any direction. The head should not tilt towards one shoulder or the other. If there is a lateral flexion of the head towards one side, and rotation of the chin towards the opposite shoulder, this is called **torticollis.** In the newborn and young infant, this is usually congenital, and represents a shortening (from fibrosis) of one side of the sternocleidomastoid muscle. The head tilts towards the shortened muscle and the chin rotates away from it. This deformity may be diagnosed at birth, but more commonly worsens during the next few weeks of life (Figure 3.4).[3]

If you find a torticollis, make sure that the cervical spine, scapulae, clavicles and upper neuro exam (including the eyes) are all normal (to exclude other causes of torticollis) e.g., a fourth nerve palsy would cause an older infant to tilt his head to compensate for his strabismus). Check for facial asymmetry, too, as this may accompany torticollis. Feel the clavicles along their entire lengths. There should be no crepitance (cracking) feeling. Clavicle fractures during the birth process are not rare.

Check the arms (at the shoulder, elbow, wrist, and hand joints) for range of motion and watch for spontaneous symmetric movement. The elbows have small flexion contractures which resolve within weeks. Birth trauma in the upper extremities can result in fractures and/or nerve damage, both of which are manifested by diminished and asymmetric upper extremity movements. Damage to the C_5 and C_6 nerve roots causes **Erb's palsy** (resulting in paralysis of the shoulder girdle and upper arm muscles). Damage to the C_7, C_8, and T1 roots results in **Klumpke's paralysis** (involving the muscles that control forearm, wrist, and hand movements). Count fingers. Examine nails and fingers for: number of joints, curvatures, webbing, and taper. Hypoplastic nails are seen in **fetal hydantoin syndrome** (associated with maternal phenytoin exposure during pregnancy). Look at the palms for the presence of a single transverse crease. These are fairly consistently found in Down syndrome but are also found in normals. Other abnormal creases and finger "whorl" patterns are distinctive but are beyond the scope of this text. Naibeds should be pink. Fingers (and toes, hands, and feet) are often blue (not the nail beds). This **acrocyanosis,** like perioral cyanosis is usually a **reflection of the newborn's normal peripheral vascular instability** and resolves over a few months.

Observe the chest again for signs of breathing difficulties.

❓ **What are the signs of dyspnea (difficulty breathing) that may be seen in the chest? . . . That's right, fast respiratory rate and retractions.**

Feel the sternum. The xiphoid may be prominent and feel somewhat distinct from the rest of the sternum. If the sternum bows in this is called a **pectus excavatum,** and if it bows out it is called a **pectus carinatum.** Usually these abnormalities are best left alone. Rarely, they need to be surgically repaired much later in childhood for cosmetic reasons.

A small amount of breast tissue will be visible and palpable (about 1 cm. in diameter) in the term infant. There may be some mild erythema and swelling and a small amount of milky discharge. This isn't present at birth but usually begins towards the end of the first week. The milky discharge is **physiologic galactorrhea.** The breast changes result from the influence of maternal hormone and resolve within a few weeks. This is not infection unless there are more extensive signs of inflammation or the baby is acting ill. In a small percentage of the population, more commonly in black infants, you may find one or more extra (accessory) nipples. These are usually found in the "milk line," along a vertical plane with the normal nipple. Some investigators feel these children are at higher risk of renal anomalies; however, there is not universal agreement concerning this risk.

If you need to measure chest circumference, it should be done at the level of the xiphoid. We don't routinely use this measurement, but it is sometimes helpful if you have concerns about either chest or head size. In the newborn, the chest circumference is usually about 2 cm. less than the head circumference. If the disparity is greater than 2 cm. you may confirm a subtle abnormality by making this comparison. As the child grows, this disparity disappears, and ultimately chest size exceeds head size.

Abdomen

Inspection of the abdomen should precede palpation. There should be no asymmetry. The newborn abdomen appears rounded convexly. Either marked concavity or distention of the belly should make you think about intra-abdominal pathology (i.e., scaphoid: diphragmatic hernia, e.g., distention: obstruction). You may choose to auscultate for bowel sounds but in a healthy newborn, particularly one who is tolerating feeds, we do not usually stop to listen.

Begin to palpate very superficially at first, allowing the infant to adjust to your stimulation, then palpate more deeply, using the same general technique you have learned on adults. The abdomen relaxes better if the baby is sucking (use a pacifier). Palpate for masses. Palpate for the liver and spleen edges. The liver edge is usually palpable, about 1–2 cm. down from the anterior costal margin, in the midclavicular line and has a firm tip. The spleen tip is either not palpable or just barely palpable. A congenital viral infection (such as rubella), may declare itself with hepatosplenomegaly (congestive heart failure may cause hepatosplenomegaly, too). If you have concerns about organomegaly or distention, you should percuss the abdomen. As you are feeling the abdomen, you may encounter a separation of the medial rectus sheath called a **diastasis recti.** A diastasis may allow a midline vertical outpouching when the baby cries; this isn't usually associated with a hernia. It is usually a normal variant and disappears in an older child.

The umbilicus, if inspected very early in life, may still be moist. If you can identify individual vessels, look for two arteries (smaller caliber and thick walled) and one vein. Variations of this (e.g., single umbilical artery) are associated with a high incidence of congenital anomalies (e.g., skeletal, gastrointestinal, renal). If there is skin laxity surrounding the umbilicus, this may represent an umbilical hernia. It will be easier to decide this when the infant is a few weeks old once the cord has fallen off. Like the diastasis recti, umbilical hernias rarely cause clinical problems, and 60% resolve in the first two years of life. The umbilical cord inserts in the midline of the abdomen. Umbilical cord insertion abnormalities that involve underlying abdominal contents (i.e., gastroschisis and omphalocele), are much more ominous than umbilical hernias. If there is herniated bowel through the abdominal wall at a site away from the umbilicus, the defect is called a **gastroschesis.** If bowel contents herniate through the umbilicus, it is called an omphalocele.

The most difficult part of the newborn abdominal exam is locating and palpating the kidneys. The most common abdominal masses in the newborn are associated with the genitourinary tract. That is one of the reasons why it is so important to palpate the kidneys. I find it easiest to use a bimanual maneuver (Figure 2.9). Place your fingers (palm side up) under the baby's back on the side you wish to examine (e.g., right fingers for the infants left side) at a level just above the iliac crest. With your free hand on the abdomen beginning medially and working laterally palpate down towards your posterior hand until you feel a firm but soft mass approximately 2 cm. wide (and as much as 4 cm. long) between your fingers. You may be able to ballot the kidney between your two hands. Perform this maneuver on both sides remembering to change hands. It takes quite a bit of practice simply to find the kidneys. Some of the time an experienced examiner cannot feel both kidneys even though they are both present. The right one is easier to feel than the left one because it's position is lower. Sometimes, even a newborn won't

cooperate for an examination. The baby may continue to cry (despite your attempts to console her) and refuse to suck on a pacifier. With each cry, her abdomen rigidly resists your efforts to get anywhere near her kidneys! One trick to attempt in this instance (also works on older children, too) is to palpate at the end of an expiration: have your hands poised on the body and ready to go. At the completion of a "wail," as the baby prepares to take a deep breath in, quickly palpate inward. With her next expiratory wail, you'll encounter resistance again. Be patient, and palpate again as the cry ends. Continue to work with her cry cycle, and eventually you'll probably feel what you've been searching for. The same technique works when palpating the rest of the abdomen.

As you move to the groin, palpate the inguinal regions and be sure you have checked for good strong femoral pulses and that there is no delay when compared simultaneously to the right brachial pulse.

Genitalia

A thorough exam in the nursery is essential for the diagnosis of congenital anomalies. Use the patient's age to your advantage, and take your time during the exam. Even though you will continue to examine the genitalia whenever you perform a complete

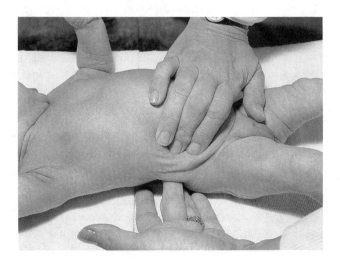

Figure 2.9. Bimanual palpation of kidney.

exam, it becomes more difficult as a child's awareness of your exam grows. **Female:** Begin with inspection of the labia. In a term infant, the labia majora cover the labia minora. As with breast tissue, there may be some swelling and erythema of the labia minora (towards the end of the first week) partly from maternal hormone. The vulva may also be swollen because of intrauterine pressure effects. Differentiate a diffusely swollen vulva from a unilateral labial mass (most likely a hernia).

Next, gently flex and abduct the thighs (Figure 2.10). With gentle lateral pressure on the labia majora you will visualize from superior to inferior: clitoris, urethra, vagina, and anus. The clitoris will seem relatively more prominent to you than in older children. Just make sure that it isn't "too" prominent! In a child with ambiguous genitalia (as in a virilized female pseudohermaphrodite with congenital adrenal hyperplasia), it won't be so easy to decide what's what! In a full term baby, the clitoris is covered by the labia when the legs are in the adducted position. If the clitoris protrudes out from the labia (and the baby isn't very thin or undergrown), the infant will need to be examined thoroughly for other signs of virilization. One example of virilization is posterior labial fusion, which obscures the

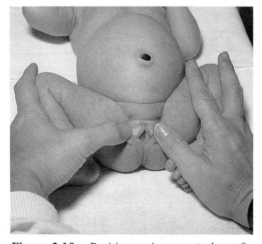

Figure 2.10.   Position to inspect newborn female genitalia.

separation of the vaginal introitus from the urethral meatus.

The next structures you encounter as you work your eyes downwards will be the pinpoint opening to the urethra, and then the vagina. Occasionally, there is a small skin tag (or two) attached to the vagina. The majority of these tags disappear under the influence of estrogen at a later age. Be certain that there is a vaginal opening, thus ruling-out vaginal agenesis. After the first few days of life, there may be a mucoid discharge and occasionally some blood from the vagina. Parents need to be informed that these effects of maternal hormones are also normal and will resolve. The anus is inspected for location and patency. An anus that is too far anterior (towards the vagina) may be associated with urologic abnormalities (there are measurement standards for normal perineal length). The anus may also have a skin tag.

Male: When examining a male, gently retract the foreskin only as far as it will easily go. Don't be surprised if it doesn't retract very much. You may be able to see the tip of the penis and the urethral opening. The term infant's penis is approximately 3–4 cm. in stretched length. If the penis has a ventral curve, this is called a **chordae.** If the urethra is situated on the dorsal (top) surface of the penis, then this is called an **epispadius,** and if it is on the ventral (underside), it is called a **hypospadius.** Defects on the glans are often, but not always associated with abnormalities of the foreskin. Urethral openings along the penile shaft proximal to the glans, or closer to the perineum will require a radiologic investigation for other GU abnormalities (these are 2nd and 3rd degrees of hypospadius). Parents are extremely sensitive about GU anomalies, so be very careful in identifying what you have found.

Next, feel the scrotum and the underlying testicles. If you cannot feel both testicles, palpate the lower abdomen carefully for masses, then proceed downwards gently along the entire length of the inguinal canal. You may find a palpable mass in the canal.

Attempt to bring the testicle down into the scrotum by using a milking or stroking action. If the testicle can be brought down into the scrotum, then the testicle is referred to as retractile. **Retractile testes** are normal. If you cannot move the testicle into the scrotum, but there is a testicle somewhere along the normal path of descent, (may not be palpable) you are dealing with an **undescended testicle.** This is also called **crypt-orchidism.** This type of testicle may or may not descend on its own. If descent has not occurred by age one year, surgical correction to bring the testicle into the scrotum will be necessary. Undescended testis and ectopic testis (abnormally placed testis outside of the normal path of descent) have a higher than normal incidence of malignant transformation and also sterility.

In the newborn, you may feel a fullness within the scrotum either on one side or both. Make sure you feel an underlying normal sized (approximately 1 cm. in length) testicle. Then use an otoscope to transilluminate the scrotum on each side. If the scrotum transilluminates clearly except for the small testicular shadow, then what you are probably feeling and seeing is a **hydrocele.** This is a fluid remnant. Most hydroceles resorb, although they are sometimes associated with an inguinal hernia. If you see a mass in the groin area, the most likely explanation is a hernia. An inguinal hernia looks like a bulge in the groin and extends above and lateral to the pubis; it may also extend into the scrotum. A hernia generally increases in size with crying or straining and decreases in size with relaxation. Scrotal transillumination may also be positive when the hernia contains bowel, thus making differentiation from a hydrocele difficult. It is helpful to remember that hydroceles are generally placed more distally, beyond the external inguinal ring. Inguinal hernias occur in both sexes but are more common in males.

The tip of the neonatal penis may be vascularly engorged and may be normally somewhat blueish, especially when exposed to the air. The scrotum over the testicles too may be blueish normally, or may be "bruised" from intrauterine pressure, (especially seen in breech presentations). While you're down there, the baby may react to your bothering him by "rewarding" you with a stream of urine. While you shriek away in surprise, don't fail to observe that he has a straight and forceful flow! Then clean everybody up . . .

Don't neglect to check for anal patency in the male too.

Lower Extremities

Proceeding downwards to examine the lower extremities (while the baby is supine), first (make sure the diaper is completely off for this . . . yes, by now you already know the "risks" of doing this . . . sorry) gently extend the legs. See if the legs are the same size (with the same muscle bulk) and length and if they look basically symmetric. Check to see that the anterior medial thigh creases are symmetrical (when you turn the baby over to examine the back, check the posterior medial thigh creases too). Asymmetry of thigh or gluteal folds should make you think of a hip abnormality, although as many as one third of normal infants have isolated thigh fold asymmetry.[4] Most newborns have flexion contractures at the hips and knees from their intrauterine position. The tibiae are usually mildly bowed laterally at their midsection (also due to fetal position). Frequently, the tibiae are also somewhat internally rotated, so that the medial malleoli are more posteriorly placed than the lateral malleoli when the knees face forwards (this becomes clinically important when children stand and walk). These findings are developmentally appropriate; it is too early in life to decide whether they will resolve.

Look at the feet. There should be no edema (as seen in Turner syndrome). If you bend down to look at the plantar surface of the foot (sole), the forefoot (toes and metatarsals) should be straight in line with the hindfoot. If so, the foot is probably normal. If the forefoot curves towards the midline, the child may have **metatarsus adductus** (Figure 2.11). Stabilize the heel between the thumb and index finger of your hand. Now try to straighten out the forefoot using the fingers of your other hand by pushing laterally against the medial curved edge (Figure 2.12). If you are able to straighten it out using moderate pressure, this deformity may correct spontaneously or with passive stretching exercises during the first two months. If it is rigid and resists straightening, or doesn't correct with passive exercise, it will require serial casting.

If the entire foot points downward (like the appearance of the foot of a horse) (Figure 2.13), and the lateral border of the foot is more distally placed than the medial border, then the child may have a clubfoot (**talipes equinovarus**). This definitely requires early orthopaedic attention.

Don't forget to count toes, and inspect for webbing, overlapping, other deformities, and restricted range of motion. Muscle tone can be assessed as you passively manipulate the legs and feet while performing your search for the congenital anomalies listed above and below. You will learn to estimate strength as you encounter kicking and opposition to some of your maneuvers; in addition when you elicit the special newborn reflexes (in the neurologic section), you will realize that intact muscle functioning is an underlying requirement for normal results.

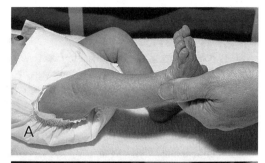

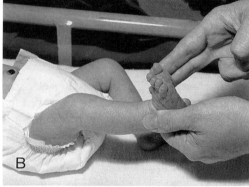

Figure 2.12A & B. To assess the severity of metatarsus adductus: stabilize the heel, then apply pressure to the forefoot.

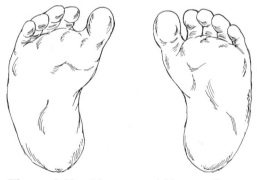

Figure 2.11. Metatarsus Adductus. Reproduced with permission. Willms JL, Lewis J. eds. Introduction to clinical medicine. Baltimore: Williams & Wilkins, 1991:140.

After you have inspected the lower extremities and manipulated the feet, return to the hips. **Congenital hip dysplasia** is one of the most difficult but important diagnoses to make in the newborn. Early treatment significantly affects prognosis. Therefore, the pediatrician must become very skilled in making this clinical diagnosis. You have already compared the lower extremities for symmetry of size, length, placement of medial thigh creases, and degree of flexion of hips and knees. Any of these might be asymmetric in unilateral hip dysplasia. To further clarify an apparent femur length inequality, flex the hips and knees, so that the heels touch the surface of the mattress. If one hip is posteriorly subluxed or dislocated, the involved femur will appear shorter, and the knee on the involved side will appear lower in height than the noninvolved side.

The maneuvers described below (Ortolani and Barlow) are the most common methods used to make the diagnosis of congenital hip

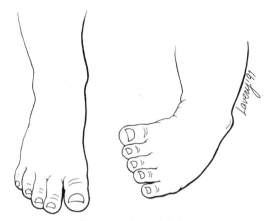

Figure 2.13. Clubfoot.

dysplasia in the newborn period. They may be performed on one hip at a time or both hips simultaneously. It is simpler to learn on one hip at a time. While standing at the "feet" end of the baby, you will use your right hand to examine her left hip and vice versa. Your nonexamining hand will stabilize the opposite hip simultaneously. After you are comfortable with the maneuvers, you may choose to examine both hips simultaneously.

Begin by examining her left hip with your right hand. First stabilize the opposite hip with your left hand. Place your left thumb on her symphysis pubis and your left fingers under her right buttock. Your right "examining" hand should bring her left hip to 90° of flexion and hold the knee fully flexed. The mid anterior tibia will rest against the palm of your hand. Place your thumb on her left anteromedial thigh just distal to the inguinal fold, and your second and third fingers on her posterolateral thigh over the greater trochanter. Gently abduct the thigh at the hip joint while lifting upwards (towards the ceiling) with your second and third fingers. This is called the **Ortolani** maneuver (Figure 2.14).

A dislocated hip may "reduce" and you will feel (or hear) either movement or a "clunk." Most of the time (in normals), you will feel nothing, or you may feel a "click," usually emanating from the knees. A click is not a true clunk (or reduction). Don't be

discouraged at this difficult distinction between a click and a clunk. Experienced pediatricians have been humbled many times over this question.

The second maneuver is the **Barlow** maneuver (Figure 2.14). This evaluates dislocatability. With your hand still wrapped around her left leg and thigh, bring the thigh back towards the midline (adduction) while pressing downwards (towards the floor) onto the anteromedial thigh with your thumb. A hip that is "dislocatable" may slide out and dislocate over the rim of the acetabulum; you may feel or hear a clunk. Repeat both maneuvers on the opposite hip.

Back

Before you dress the baby, turn her over and look closely at her back and the posterior

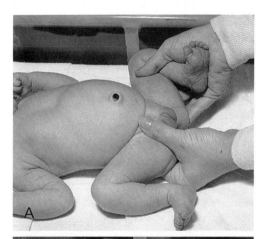

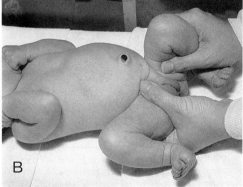

Figure 2.14. The Ortolani and Barlow maneuvers.

aspects of her legs. The spine should appear straight and scapulae and iliac crests should be symmetric. Palpate the spine along it's full length and feel the bottom of the sacrum. Note **any** lesions (e.g., soft tissue masses, hair tufts, hemangiomas, etc.) or skin defects (even dimples) overlying the spine. Dimples over the lower spine are common and are usually not significant (as long as the dimple isn't really the superficial manifestation of a skin defect or sinus tract). If you are able to spread the skin apart to see that the skin is intact under a dimple, then there isn't likely to be an underlying problem. However, any lesion over the spine (especially masses) should receive some evaluation for an underlying abnormality of neural tube development.

If you see a **black and blue** macule or patch (this is most common over the lower spine and buttocks, but is also found in the shoulder region) you have identified a **mongolian spot.** This is not another bruise from birth. It is seen more in dark-skinned children. This is a normal variant with absolutely no clinical significance and usually fades over time. This spot has no relationship to Down syndrome.

Skin

As long as the baby is still in her "birthday suit," complete your assessment of the skin. Evaluate her overall color (e.g., look for jaundice, true cyanosis, pallor).

❓ In the newborn, where does jaundice first manifest itself? Yes, in the face. As the serum bilirubin rises, jaundice progresses caudally towards the feet.

Occasionally a baby will look very ruddy. This sometimes represents underlying polycythemia. Another baby might demonstrate a sharp vertical demarcation down the center of the body with one side of the body appearing redder than the other. This is called a **harlequin color change** and, like acrocyanosis, reflects the temporary and nonpathologic vascular instability of the neonate.

She may still have some fetal **vernix** (means varnish in Latin) **caseosa** (means cheesy in Latin) in her skin folds and nail beds. This fetal covering consists of sebum and desquamated epithelial cells. Most of the **lanugo** (fetal hair) has been shed prior to term. If you see cracking or desquamation, do not assume that she will be destined to have dry skin. This is a very common misconception. In the term infant some skin peeling is always normal. If there is an excess of peeling, she may be postmature (more about that in a little while). You may have already found some milia on her face.

❓ What are milia? Good, they are harmless retention cysts or papules!

You may find some hemangiomas. The common ones are:

Stork bites (or **salmon patches**) (Figure 2.15) are very superficial, pink to red, flat lesions, which are present at birth mostly over the eyelids, nasal bridge, and nape of neck. These fade during a period of months to years (the neck nevus tends to fade less completely).

Strawberry hemangiomas (Figure 2.16) (called strawberries because of their bumpy, red surfaces) may be found anywhere on the body. This type of capillary hemangioma is not usually visible at birth; however, with

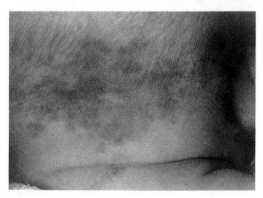

Figure 2.15. Stork bite on the nape of the neck. Reproduced with permission. Hurwitz S. Clinical pediatric dermatology. Philadelphia: W.B. Saunders, 1981:195. Courtesy Sidney Hurwitz, M.D.

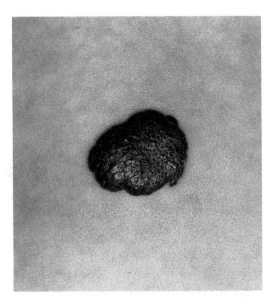

Figure 2.16. Strawberry hemangioma. Reproduced with permission. Hurwitz S. Clinical pediatric dermatology. Philadelphia, W.B. Saunders: 1981:191. Courtesy Sidney Hurwitz, M.D.

very careful inspection, you may find its forerunner: a circumscribed, hypovascularized area with telangiectasias or tiny red threads within it. The characteristic well-demarcated strawberry then appears within weeks of birth, and grows rapidly in size and palpability during the first year. During the toddler and school years it involutes, almost always completely. Raised hemangiomas are important to follow if they are very large because they may cause troublesome bleeding or platelet trapping. It is also important to closely follow hemangiomas that are near the eyes, nares, mouth, or trachea, because as they grow, they may interfere with a vital function. Parents worry a lot about these hemangiomas; but, unless there are problems of bleeding or encroachment, they can be reassured as to the benign prognosis.

Port wine stains (Figure 2.17) are present at birth. These are flat hemangiomas which are red or pink at birth but which eventually darken to a deep red or purple. They grow in proportion to the child. Unlike the stork bite, these do not fade and, therefore, may be quite disfiguring. Port wine stains tend to be unilateral; they may

be found anywhere on the body but are most common over the face or neck. If this type of hemangioma involves the area of the face innervated by the ophthalmic division of the trigeminal nerve, the baby may have **Sturge-Weber** syndrome (with cerebral vascular abnormalities and possible mental retardation, seizures, motor, and ophthalmologic problems).

Note the presence of all birthmarks. Measure and describe them, remembering to include a statement about color (including hypopigmentation). Isolated **cafe-au-lait spots** (flat, oval tan lesions with distinct borders) and **depigmented spots** may be present at birth in normal individuals; they may also be the first manifestation of a neurocutaneous disorder such as neurofibromatosis and tuberous sclerosis. In an otherwise normal newborn, without a family history of these disorders, we note the presence of these lesions and maintain a

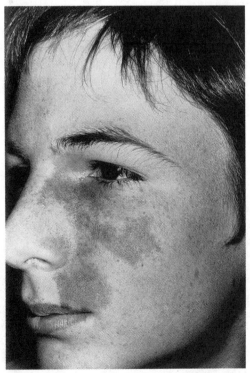

Figure 2.17. Port wine stain. Reproduced with permission. Hurwitz S. Clinical pediatric dermatology. Philadelphia: W.B. Saunders, 1981:195. Courtesy Sidney Hurwitz, M.D.

slightly higher than average vigilance for any further manifestations of these disorders (see Figures 4.1, 4.2).

A final note about some acquired rashes.

The most common newborn rash is called **erythema toxicum** (Figure 2.18). It has a "flea-bite" appearance with scattered erythematous macules (with a predilection for trunk, face, and extremities, not the palms and soles), sometimes with papulo-pustular centers. These benign lesions "come and go" during the first two weeks of life. They require no treatment.

You might also see **miliaria rubra,** (not to be confused with milia) which is due to obstruction of sweat glands. This condition is characterized by tiny papules or vesicles, sometimes with an erythematous halo base most commonly noted on the face and neck. This is also self resolving. Miliaria rubra is commonly referred to as "heat rash."

A third benign rash (seen much more commonly in black neonates) is: **transient neonatal pustular melanosis** (Figure 2.19) (remembering the name is harder than remembering the rash!). Vesiculopustules can be present anywhere (including palms and soles) at birth. Within a few days these rupture. Some of the lesions will leave behind pigmented macules with a fine scale surrounding them. Resolution is ultimately complete.

When we are unable to decide about

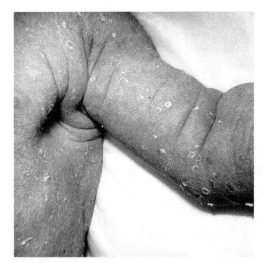

Figure 2.19. TNPM: Transient neonatal pustular melanosis. Photo courtesy of Stanley F. Glazer, M.D.

whether or not pustular lesions with surrounding erythema represent one of the benign rashes or the more worrisome staph aureus, then we gram stain and culture the pustule contents. The same is true for vesicles (in this case, we would also perform cytology to look for "giant" cells associated with herpes). The vesicles associated with herpes simplex usually appear after the first few days of life (but may be present at birth). If these are present, the baby may become very ill.

Neurologic and Development

The neurologic component completes your exam. You already have a **general sense** about this baby. You should consider her state of arousal, the fluidity and spontaneity of her movements, and her posture at rest. At rest, the term infant will be partially "flexed" at the elbows, hips, and knees.

When you move her about, does she startle very easily, cry excessively (or with a high pitch?) or develop **sustained** leg or facial clonus? We call this type of baby "jittery." Occasional and short (a few beats) clonus isn't abnormal in the newborn. She may have underlying central nervous system pathology or a systemic infection. The other type of worrisome (full term) baby is not

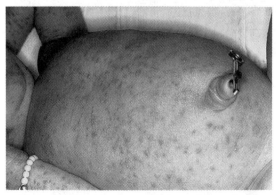

Figure 2.18. Erythema Toxicum. Reproduced with permission. Hurwitz S. Clinical pediatric dermatology. Philadelphia: W.B. Saunders, 1981:11. Courtesy Sidney Hurwitz, M.D.

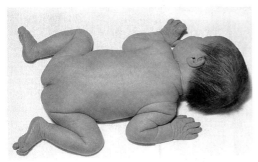

Figure 2.20. Flexed posture of the term newborn.

naturally flexed and feels like a "limp dish rag" when you pick her up.

The rest of the neonatal neurologic exam follows the same general outline as in older children, but because of the absence of voluntary cooperation, some of the maneuvers are different. A few components are nearly impossible to evaluate in newborns (e.g., cranial nerve I). In addition, because the nervous system is still very immature, some of the findings in normal newborns are quite unique to this age group.

Start with the face and review the **cranial nerves (II–XII)**. You performed most of these maneuvers as you proceeded through your general exam. You observed her blink in response to bright light **(II)**, examined the fundus (red reflex) **(II)**; if she was cooperative, she focused on, and tracked an object **(II)**. You observed her pupillary response to light **(III)** and observed her conjugate eye movements in all directions of gaze III, IV, VI). You checked for doll's eyes **(III, IV, VI and the vestibular component of VIII)** and for the absence of ptosis **(III)**.

❓ By what age should occasional, normal, disconjugate eye movements disappear (if there is no strabismus)? Good! By age three months.

To evaluate the sensory component of V (corneal reflex), blow gently on her face and watch her blink (don't do this if you have a cold). You felt her mouth close securely while sucking **(motor V)**; and observed her

facial expression (eye closure and symmetry of facial creases) during crying **(motor VII)**. To grossly assess hearing **(VIII)**, introduce a novel sound (e.g., a bell), and watch her "alert" by quieting her movements and opening her eyes. If she's feeding well, it's likely that her swallowing is effective **(IX and X)**, and her gag is intact **(IX)**, and her tongue movements are strong **(XII)**. Cranial nerve **XI** is difficult to evaluate in newborns; however, in the absence of torticollis, it is unlikely to be abnormal.

Sensation is a little difficult to evaluate in newborns. It can be done by testing withdrawal to light stroking or pin prick if necessary.

Her deep tendon reflexes will seem a little brisk to you (about a 3 out of 4 response). As we have mentioned, she may have a few (1–2) beats of clonus on either or both sides. On the opposite end of the spectrum, a small percentage of normal newborns will have apparent decreased or absent DTRs. The plantar reflex may not give you any information at this age, as both flexion and extension of the toes may be seen in normal newborns.

There are some special newborn reflexes which give information about the general integrity of the neurologic system. To test for the **Moro reflex** (Figure 2.21) cradle her head and upper back in your hands and forearms (while she is supine). Then allow her head to fall back with your hands as you abruptly (but gently) move your hands back towards the surface of the bassinet. The normal response is a symmetric abduction of the arms with extension of the fingers (and some lesser abduction of the legs) followed by a return to the usual flexion posture.

A "complete" Moro tells you also that the brain, the nerves, and muscles are working together. In addition, if she has an arm paralysis or fracture, there will be an asymmetric moro. This reflex sometimes triggers a few beats of unsustained clonus of the arms or legs which are normal at this age.

A second reflex is called **placing and stepping.** This is fun to show parents. Pick her up with your hands under her axillae and

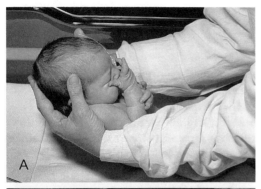

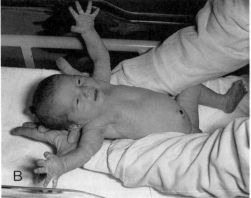

Figure 2.21A & B.   The Moro reflex

hold her upright. Then gently scrape the top of her foot along the underside of a table or bassinet edge. She will respond by flexing then extending her leg (that is placing). When the sole of her foot touches a flat surface, she will "walk" for you! (That is stepping).

You can also show parents her **reflex grasp** by placing a finger in her palm. She will close her fingers around yours.

You have already made a lot of observations about the motor components of the neurologic examination. The flexed posture of the full term baby (vs the extended posture of a premature) give you information about tone and symmetry (the extremities of hypotonic infants may also not be flexed at rest). The special newborn reflexes allow observations of function and symmetry of large muscle groups. In addition, muscle bulk, strength, and tone should be

assessed as you handle your patient. One way to learn what is normal is to examine a lot of newborns. In addition, to assess tone, you may pull her up gently from the supine position by grasping her hands in yours. The full term baby's head will not remain totally extended as you pull her to a sitting position but instead may begin to flex slightly as her head comes off the mattress. The hypotonic infant (and more premature infant) will have no head flexion during this maneuver. In addition, if you place her belly down and then pick her up around the middle, her **ventral suspension** will look like this (Figure 2.22):

She should not roll into a complete circle. Some newborns can even pick their heads up a little from the prone position.

In addition, when you support the baby in an upright position by placing your hands in her axillae, the newborn with normal tone and strength should not **"slip through"** your hands (or be totally supported by you); you shouldn't have to hold the baby upright, just support her.

Now you have finished with the routine exam of the newborn. This took quite bit of time to work through together. In practice, it will go much faster, especially now that you understand how and why we do each maneuver. If you follow the same sequence every time, you are less likely to omit something important.

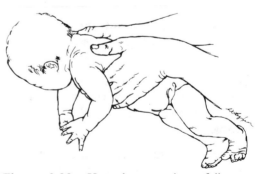

Figure 2.22. Ventral suspension: full-term newborn. Reproduced with permission. Willms JL, Lewis J. Introduction to clinical medicine. Baltimore: Williams & Wilkins, 1991:137.

GESTATIONAL AGE AND APPROPRIATENESS OF SIZE FOR GESTATIONAL AGE

Student Tasks

1. Determine gestational age.
2. Determine appropriateness of size for gestational age.

Gestational Age

Now it is time to organize some of the information you have obtained. During your early nursery experiences, you will probably work most closely with full-term or near-term infants. However some of the time you will examine an infant who because of size, appearance, or behavior doesn't quite fit with your expectations for a full-term baby. Maternal dates and prenatal ultrasound may be inaccurate or unavailable. You will need to know how to determine gestational age by physical exam. Important clinical decisions often depend on this assessment. Infants are categorized into three groups based on their gestational age: 1) **Premature:** 37 weeks gestation or less; 2) **Full-term:** 38 to 42 weeks; 3) **Postmature:** greater than 42 weeks gestation.

Estimation of gestational age utilizes findings on two types of rating scales: neuromuscular maturity and physical maturity. The principle behind both scales is that certain physical attributes and neurologic findings evolve in a predictable and progressive fashion through the latter half of gestation. There are several versions of each type of scale and rating system. Some methods use only one type of scale, and others use both. Values on each scale are assigned to specific findings and the totals are added. Total scores correspond to certain gestational ages. The numbers aren't important, just the general principles.

Physical maturity scales include external physical findings which are assessed by inspection and palpation (e.g., thickness of skin, extent of plantar surface of the foot covered by creases, appearance of genitalia). Physical maturity is most accurately assessed

as soon after birth as feasible. The **"premie"** may be recognized as having: little or no palpable breast tissue, little or no creases on the sole of the foot, skin that is smooth with veins that are visible, and ear pinnae that are pliable and rudimentary. The **term** infant has palpable breast tissue, creases over the entire sole, thicker pink skin, and firm pinnae with well-defined folds. The **postmature** infant displays physical characteristics which have progressed further along the continuum: the skin is leathery, cracked, wrinkled, and devoid of lanugo, nails are long, and soles have deep creases.

Neuromuscular maturity scales include assessments of passive tone and posture. Neuromuscular maturity is optimally assessed when the infant is quiet and rested. If the baby is depressed (e.g., because of birth asphyxia or maternal sedation) the findings may not accurately reflect gestational age. In this case, the neuromuscular assessment may need to be repeated during the second or third day of life. The **premie** is **floppy and flexible.** At rest, she lies with her extremities in extension, or all stretched out. When she is suspended prone in the air with the examiner supporting her chin she is very floppy; she almost forms a circle with her head and body (Figure 2.23).

When she is pulled by the wrists from supine to sitting, she has little or no evidence of head support. Her flexibility is demonstrated by a variety of maneuvers which include the "heel to ear" maneuver (see Figure 2.24) and the "scarf sign," (see Figure 2.25). When these maneuvers are performed on the most premature infant, the heel reaches all the way to the ear, and the elbow reaches the opposite anterior axillary line.

We have previously described the posture and tone of the **term** infant: the extremities are held in flexion, and some head control is demonstrated on ventral suspension and pull to sitting. The "heel to ear" and "scarf sign" maneuvers demonstrate that the term infant isn't nearly as flexible as a premie. That is, the heel may only reach as far as the

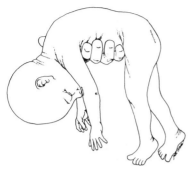

Figure 2.23. Ventral suspension: premature newborn. Reproduced with permission. Willms JL, Lewis J. Introduction to clinical medicine. Baltimore: Williams & Wilkins, 1991:137.

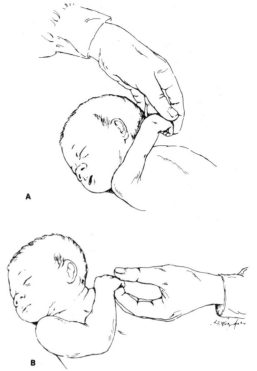

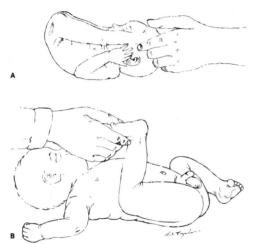

Figure 2.24. Heel-to-ear maneuver: while the infant is supine, the examiner holds the baby's foot in one hand and moves it up as close to the head as possible without forcing it. At the same time the pelvis is held flat on the table. Reproduced with permission. Willms JL, Lewis J. Introduction to clinical medicine. Baltimore: Williams & Wilkins, 1991:136.
>   **Figure 2.24A.**   Premature newborn.
>   **Figure 2.24B.**   Full-term newborn.

Figure 2.25. Scarf sign maneuver: while the infant is supine, the examiner grasps the infant's hand and draws it across the infant's neck as far to the opposite shoulder as it will go. (The elbow may be lifted across the body.) Reproduced with permission. Willms JL, Lewis J. Introduction to clinical medicine. Baltimore: Williams & Wilkins, 1991:135.
>   **Figure 2.25A.**   Premature newborn.
>   **Figure 2.25B.**   Full-term newborn.

umbilicus, and the elbow may not even reach the midline of the thorax. The **post-mature** infant will demonstrate all of the neurologic criteria on the mature end of the scale, with less exceptions than a full-term might demonstrate.

The Newborn Maturity Rating used at many institutions is found below (Figure 2.26).[5] This scoring system, devised by Ballard et al., is an abbreviated version of that originally devised by Dubowitz and colleagues. Dubowitz et al based their scoring system on the neurologic findings of Amiel-Tison and the physical characteristics described by Farr et al.[6,7,8]. The clinician often refers to this process of scoring gestational age as performing a "**Dubowitz.**"

Your instructors will demonstrate the rest of the neuromuscular maneuvers. In addition, a rough estimate of maturity may be obtained by doubling the physical maturity score.

Appropriateness of Size for Gestational Age

Now that you have a basic idea of how mature your baby is, look at the newborn

NEUROMUSCULAR MATURITY

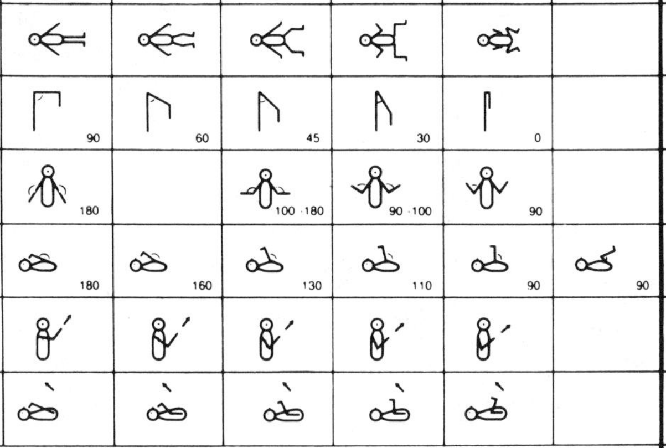

NEUROMUSCULAR MATURITY SIGN	SCORE 0	1	2	3	4	5	RECORD SCORE HERE
POSTURE							
SQUARE WINDOW (WRIST)	90	60	45	30	0		
ARM RECOIL	180	100-180	90-100	90			
POPLITEAL ANGLE	180	160	130	110	90	90	
SCARF SIGN							
HEEL TO EAR							

TOTAL NEUROMUSCULAR MATURITY SCORE

SCORE

Neuromuscular _____

Physical _____

Total _____

MATURITY RATING

TOTAL MATURITY SCORE	GESTATIONAL AGE (WEEKS)
5	26
10	28
15	30
20	32
25	34
30	36
35	38
40	40
45	42
50	44

PHYSICAL MATURITY

PHYSICAL MATURITY SIGN	SCORE 0	1	2	3	4	5	RECORD SCORE HERE
SKIN	gelatinous red, transparent	smooth pink, visible veins	superficial peeling, & or rash few veins	cracking pale area rare veins	parchment deep cracking no vessels	leathery cracked wrinkled	
LANUGO	none	abundant	thinning	bald areas	mostly bald		
PLANTAR CREASES	no crease	faint red marks	anterior transverse crease only	creases ant 2 3	creases cover entire sole		
BREAST	barely percept.	flat areola no bud	stippled areola. 1-2mm bud	raised areola. 3-4mm bud	full areola 5-10mm bud		
EAR	pinna flat. stays folded	sl. curved pinna; soft with slow recoil	well-curv. pinna; soft but ready recoil	formed & firm with instant recoil	thick cartilage ear stiff		
GENITALS (Male)	scrotum empty no rugae		testes descending. few rugae	testes down good rugae	testes pendulous deep rugae		
GENITALS (Female)	prominent clitoris & labia minora		majora & minora equally prominent	majora large. minora small	clitoris & minora completely covered		

TOTAL PHYSICAL MATURITY SCORE

GESTATIONAL AGE (weeks)

By dates _____

By ultrasound _____

By score _____

Figure 2.26. Scoring system for clinical assessment of fetal maturation in newborn infants. Used with permission. Ballard JL, Novak KK, Driver M. A simplified score for assessment of fetal maturation of newly born infants. J Pediatr 1979;95:769–774.

growth charts in the Appendix. Most of you will have decided that your baby is approximately term gestation. Plot the weight, length, and head circumference on the growth charts under the appropriate gestational age. You will notice that each measurement falls in one of three areas: **AGA** (appropriate for gestational age), **SGA** (small for gestational age), **LGA** (large for gestational age). A mature (full term) baby, who is absolutely normal, will be appropriate for gestational age (the real meaning of this is . . . not too small and not too big). If you discover that this mature, full-term baby is small for gestational age or SGA (e.g., a full-term baby who weighs 4 lbs. and is only 17 inches long), then you have discovered that somewhere along the line there may have been an in utero problem. SGA and LGA babies, whatever the gestational age have a higher incidence of certain in utero and postnatal problems. You will learn more specifics as you go along in pediatrics. Some common examples of SGA (or growth retarded) babies are those with congenital viral infections and infants of alcoholic mothers. The LGA baby is often large for either familial or unknown reasons. If there is a pathologic cause, it's most common association is maternal diabetes.

Now that you know where your baby "plots out," you've gotten more confirmation of whether or not this is truly a perfectly "fine" newborn. Now, review the records to locate the baby's Apgar scores. You will probably find them recorded on the copy of the mother's delivery sheet in the baby's chart.

THE APGAR SCORING SYSTEM

Student Task

1. List the components of the Apgar scoring system.

The Apgar scoring system was developed by Dr. Virginia Apgar, an anesthesiologist from New Jersey, to help evaluate how successfully the fetus manages the immediate transition to newborn life. It is used in every delivery room by whomever (nurse, physi-

cian) is responsible for "receiving" the infant after delivery. Sometimes the obstetrician does the scoring. It is important for you to understand this scoring for several reasons. First, it provides information about the initial stability of the infant. Second, it is sometimes used for prognostic information (although one should be very cautious about this). Third, many parents will want to know the results of their child's "first test." Just be careful not to fall into the trap of equating the numbers, particularly the one- and five-minute score, with longterm significance. A low ten minute score has been associated with a higher (than average) incidence of lonterm neurologic sequelae. The final reason you should understand this score is that this is the baby's first encounter with a type of "physical exam," and by the end of this chapter, you will be skilled in all of the "newborn exams!"

When you spend time in the delivery room, you will learn exactly how to determine this score. It is performed at one minute and five minutes after birth. If a baby is doing poorly, it will be done again at ten minutes. The numbers obtained in the appropriate categories are added up to a possible total of ten. You can feel reassured (and so can parents), that most babies do not "get a 10," because a point has been taken off for color.

Table 2.1
The Apgar Scoring System

Criterion	Score		
	2	1	0
Heart rate	>100	<100	absent
Respiratory Effort	good crying	weak cry hypoventilation	absent
Reflex Irritability (response of skin stimulation to feet)	cry	some motion	no response
Muscle tone	well-flexed	some flexion of extremities	limp
Color	completely pink	body pink extremities blue	blue, pale

❓ What is the significance of bluish extremity (not nailbed) color in newborns??? . . . Good, you were paying attention! The peripheral extremities can be bluish for quite a while, or off and on, particularly with crying!

A pneumonic to remember APGAR is: **A** = appearance (skin color), **P** = pulse, **G** = grimace (reflex irritability), **A** = activity, and **R** = respiration.

A score of 8–10 is excellent; 4–7 is worrisome, and 0–3 is critical.

Now, you've "got your data," and it's time to meet mom (or mom and dad). Remember to look at both parents for "family" characteristics. It's now important to observe the interactions between parents and baby. Ask the nursery nurse where mom's room is . . .

THE PRENATAL AND PERINATAL HISTORY

Student Task

1. Obtain a prenatal and perinatal history from the mother (or parents).

As you enter the mom's room, be cautious. Knock first, identify yourself, and ask if it's o.k. to come in. Not infrequently, she will be in the midst of having a dressing changed, trying to go to the bathroom, or talking on the phone. Once she's free, she will probably welcome your visit. Explain that you have just examined her baby and would like to tell her about the exam. Congratulate her! Tell her what a good job she has done. You can then add that you would also like to review the prenatal history with her. If you explain that this information will be helpful in taking care of her baby, she will probably respond very positively.

If you (as in most cases) have found that her baby has a normal physical exam, tell her right away. This is reassuring and sets a positive tone for your interview. As a student, you will not be the initial bearer of bad news.

While you are with her, observe her mood and interest in hearing about the baby. Does she ask questions about her? If you have brought the baby out with you, observe how she interacts with her: Does she touch her?, hold and cuddle her closely?, look at her?, speak endearingly to her? If so, then you have positive information that she is forming a strong attachment to her infant. Assuming mom isn't experiencing a lot of pain (or under the influence of narcotics or sedatives), if the answers to the above questions are negative, concern about her psychologic state or bonding should be raised. If dad is present, try to make the same observations about him.

While you are observing, ask for the substance of the prenatal history. Start with an open-ended question such as: How was this pregnancy? You can become more specific as you go along. While this seems like a lot of information to obtain, with practice you will be able to do it in just a few minutes. The specific order is not important. Many of the answers (especially family and social history) will come out in general conversation.

Some of the details (e.g., labor and delivery meds, problems) may need to be obtained directly from the mother's chart. In addition, you may feel uncomfortable about pursuing some of the details (e.g., reasons for prior abortions or miscarriages) at a time when you are attempting to be positive about this new and normal infant. There are two ways to approach this problem. One approach is to omit these direct questions and obtain this information from the chart too. Another way (usually my approach) is to ask for this information using a "matter of fact" manner, couching questions within a larger body of many other "routine" pregnancy and health related questions. This approach works for me because I have practiced it many times over. It also works because I usually obtain prenatal history from **two** sources: from the mother's chart **and** from the mother. Approaching it this way increases the chance that the history is accurate and forewarns me to approach certain questions delicately or avoid them if they aren't pertinent.

Pregnancy Maternal **age, EDC** (due date); **G** (gravida status-# of pregnancies); **P** (para status-# of potentially viable infants delivered); **Ab** (abortus status-# of miscarriages/abortions); medical **complications** during this pregnancy (e.g., bleeding, infections, hypertension, diabetes, excessive or small weight gain) and **therapies** necessary for these complications; **other medication** taken during pregnancy; maternal **smoking, alcohol consumption, other substance abuse** (extent, frequency, timing). Was this **pregnancy planned?** Did she have **prenatal care?** What method is planned for feeding (**breast or bottle**)?

Labor and delivery Was **labor spontaneous or induced** (length of labor, reason for induction)? Amniotic **membranes ruptured** when? Fluid **meconium stained? Medicines** during labor and delivery? **Delivery mode** (reason for cesarean section)? Newborn **presentation** (vertex, breech)? Newborn **Apgar scores?** Condition of **newborn in delivery room** (delivery room intervention required)? How does she **feel about her labor and delivery?**

Past medical history **Significant** past or present nonpregnancy related **health problems.** Attempt to determine if mother has any **HIV** risk factors (e.g., intravenous drug use past or present, history of blood or blood product transfusions, sexual partner of someone with HIV risk); **hepatitis B** history; **herpes** history.

Family history Inquire about the **health** status of **other immediate family** members. Are there **any** family members with **congenital anomalies** or other potentially inherited medical problems?

Social history Inquire about the **home environment.** For example, who lives at home? If parents unmarried, is father of baby involved? Do mother or father work outside the home (financial resources adequate? childcare arrangements planned?)

How do parents and siblings feel about baby (concerns and fears)? Name of pediatrician? Is home physically ready for baby (crib, car seat)? For male infants, is circumcision planned?

Now you have the tools to continue the process of substantive learning about the newborn. Recording the information you have gathered is also important. As you read through the form that follows, you will be pleasantly surprised at the level of expertise you have attained!

WRITTEN RECORD FOR THE PRENATAL HISTORY AND NEWBORN PHYSICAL EXAM
Student Task

1. Record the prenatal history and newborn physical exam.

On the following page is an example of the form presently in use in our hospital. It assumes you have performed a complete newborn history and physical examination. While it does not ask for a description of every finding, there is room to record anything of significance.

THE PROBLEM: "DOCTOR, THIS BABY DOESN'T LOOK RIGHT!"

January 20

It is 3:15 p.m. You have been busy in the outpatient department seeing children with earaches and sore throats. The atmosphere is harried as the afternoon is filling up with last minute calls for emergency appointments. Your senior resident, John, looks over the pile of charts of waiting children and sighs. Just then the phone rings. It is the head nurse in the newborn nursery. She is concerned about B.G. (baby girl) Stone who was born one hour ago. The baby has a low temperature and is showing signs of respiratory distress. Your resident sighs again, wonders what time he will ever be finished for the day and says, "We'd better get upstairs quickly."

On your way upstairs, you review the newborn history and physical in your mind. Just then, your resident asks if you remember the signs of respiratory distress.

❓ **What are the signs of respiratory distress in the newborn? . . . Good, you remembered!: Consistent tachypnea >60 breaths**

ADMISSION-DISCHARGE EXAMINATION

Patient Identification

Birth Date: _____ Time: _____ ☐ AM ☐ PM Private Physician: _____ Obstetrician: _____

PRENATAL HISTORY
Mother:
G: _____ P: _____ Ab: _____ Age: _____ Blood Type: _____ Serology: _____ EDC: _____
Pregnancy Complications: _____

Delivery Mode & Complications: _____

Apgar: 1': _____ 5' _____
Medical Problems: _____

Pertinent Social History: _____

Pertinent Family History: _____

Admission Examination	Discharge Examination
Wt: (lbs.) Lgt: (in.) HC: (cm)	Wt: (lbs.) Lgt: (in.) HC: (cm)

	WNL	(If abnormal, describe)		WNL	(If abnormal, describe)
Skin Clear?	☐		Skin:	☐	_____
(Note jaundice/cyanosis/rash)		_____			_____
Head			Head:	☐	_____
Fontanelles palpable/normal?	☐	_____			_____
Sutures OK?	☐	_____			
(note significant molding/caput)					
Eyes			Eyes:	☐	_____
Red Reflex present?	☐	_____			_____
Conjunctiva clear?	☐	_____			
Ears			Ears:	☐	_____
Position & shape normal?	☐	_____			
Cartilage present?	☐	_____			
Nose patent?	☐	_____	Nose:	☐	_____
Mouth					
Palate intact?	☐	_____	Mouth:	☐	_____
Neck					
Clavicles intact?	☐	_____	Neck:	☐	_____
Chest					
Breast tissue palpable?	☐	_____	Chest:	☐	_____
Lungs					
Clear?	☐	_____	Lungs:	☐	_____
Heart					
Rate/Rhythm normal?	☐	_____	Heart:	☐	_____
Murmur absent?	☐	_____			
Pulses adequate?	☐	_____			
Abdomen			Abdomen:	☐	_____
Organomegaly/masses absent?	☐	_____			_____
Anus patent?	☐	_____			_____
Cord vessels normal?	☐	_____			
Genitalia			Genitalia:	☐	_____
Normal ♂ or ♀?	☐	_____			_____
Testicles ↓↓?	☐	_____			_____
Hernia/Hydrocele absent?	☐	_____			
Musculoskeletal			Musculoskeletal:	☐	_____
Hips in place?	☐	_____			_____
Digits all present?	☐	_____			_____
Neurological			Neurological:	☐	_____
Strong moro/suck/root?	☐	_____			_____
Good grasp/tone?	☐	_____			_____

Term: ☐   Preterm: ☐   Post Term: ☐   AGA: SGA: LGA:
Plan:

_____ M.D.
Date   Physician

Assessment/Plan:

_____ M.D.
Date   Physician

Figure 2.27. Newborn Physical Examination and Prenatal History.

per minute, retractions, nasal flaring, and grunting.

When you enter the nursery, (Did you remember to wash your hands and grab a stethoscope?) Patty, the charge nurse, looks worried. John heads for the baby's warmer and asks Patty if she knows any of the prenatal history.

❓ Can you remember some of the questions to ask in the prenatal history? Where can you find some of this information before you see mom? . . . The delivery sheet (a copy of which should be in the nursery), the footprint sheet, nurses notes, and mother's chart . . . Great!

Patty pulls out the delivery sheet and you review it at the baby's bedside:
Susan Stone Age: 28 G1 P1 Ab0 EDC February 1
Pregnancy: no complications
Onset of labor: spontaneous, 4 hours prior to delivery
Medications during labor: none
Rupture of membranes: 2 hours prior to delivery, fluid clear
Delivery: vaginal, vertex presentation
Apgars: 1 minute: 8; 5 minutes: 8
B.G. Stone: Birth Weight: 4 lbs. 7 ounces (2000 gms.)
Birth Length: 17 ½ inches (45 cm)

❓ Think about this information for a moment. (Hint, you may want to look at the charts in the Appendix) . . . Yes! There is definitely something that doesn't jive. This is not a "regular" full term baby. This baby is obviously small. Is she premature or full term? Well, you now know that the only way to answer that is to examine her.

Your resident stands by while you examine her. On exam you find: her eyes are closed. There are few spontaneous momements. Respiratory rate: 70. You hear a soft grunt on expiration and observe mild nasal flaring. Heart rate: 180, rate regular. A soft blowing systolic murmur is present along the left sternal border at the 2nd left intercostal space. There are no other pathologic sounds. The precordium does not feel hyperdynamic; the pulses aren't weak or bounding. There are no retractions. The breath sounds are bronchovesicular, without crackles or other patho-

logic sounds. As you examine her, she begins to stir and cry weakly. When you return to the rest of the "head to toe" exam, you do not note any dysmorphic features. Her head circumference measures 31 cm.

❓ What other information (besides the chest exam) will be helpful in deciding how much respiratory distress is present? . . . That's it! . . . Her coloring . . . Her extremities are bluish . . . Does that concern you? Not necessarily. There is some mild perioral cyanosis, too. But her lips, mucous membranes, and nail beds are pink.

Her rectal temperature is 96.8 F. (She is cold!)
Finally you perform a very rapid assessment of her gestational age: You find: skin is smooth with a small amount of superficial peeling. There is the bare beginning of a breast bud; the pinnae are soft, easily folded, but return to correct position when folded; and there is one transverse crease on the sole. Ah ha! This certainly confirms what you suspected! This baby is premature (34 weeks by exam). Now plot her weight, height, and head circumference on the newborn growth charts in the Appendix. What do you find? That's right. This baby is AGA (appropriate for gestational age) in all dimensions. That's reassuring.

Recall your introduction to the nursery. Remember what we said about temperature control? Correct. Some prematures have trouble regulating their body temperatures. Baby girl Stone is a 34-week, appropriate for gestational age, baby who is showing some mild respiratory distress and is "cold." Now it's time for me to help you a little:

Some babies breathe fast initially because they are cold. Sometimes the respiratory distress and the temperature instability signal a more serious problem such as: hyaline membrane disease, sepsis, or hypoglycemia. As you progress in pediatrics, you will learn more about how to decide what's going on and what to do about these problems. Unlike older infants, true fever is rare in newborns, and if present at birth may reflect mother's temperature rather than baby's.

John quickly orders a Dextro-stix (to estimate her blood glucose), some lab studies and a chest x-ray. He also turns the temperature control up on the warmer in order to raise the baby's own temperature back to normal. You both go to the recovery room to speak with the parents.

John greets the Stones, introduces you and

appraises them of the situation. Remember, this is your first opportunity to observe for parental affect and attachment! The Stones are appropriately anxious. John describes the situation to them. He shares some of his concerns about their daughter but also emphasizes the normal features of her exam.

You review the prenatal history with them.

This was Mrs. Stone's first pregnancy. She had no medical complications. Her periods have always been irregular. The couple had been trying to conceive for about a year before Mrs. Stone realized she might be pregnant. She had several "false alarms" for a few months. By the time her pregnancy test was positive, she was no longer sure when her last "real" menstrual period was. The EDC listed on the delivery sheet was a "best guess" by the parents, confirmed by a single ultrasound during the second trimester. John confirms that the baby is premature. You obtain the rest of the history, which does not add any additional or worrisome information. Then it is time to go back and check on the baby and the lab tests.

When you return to the nursery, Patty looks relieved. The baby's temperature is normal. The respiratory rate is 50. She has stopped grunting. You examine her and she is sleeping peacefully. The initial lab tests and chest x-ray are normal . . . John concludes that she had the expected temperature instability of the premature. It is unlikely, now that her physical exam is normal, that there is something more serious occurring. She will be watched very closely for the next 24 hours. Now, she will be moved to an incubator where she will stay until she can regulate her own temperature in an open bassinet. John writes some orders and then you return to the recovery room to reassure the Stones.

Even though you have not yet acquired the substantive knowledge to diagnose definitively or treat a newborn, you have come a long way! With your history and physical skills, you have been able to take the first crucial steps in the management process! You have also learned one additional axiom: don't assume that the information you receive second hand is always correct!

References

1. Hall JG. When a child is born with congenital anomalies. Contemp Pediatr 1988;8:79.
2. Cloutier M. Pulmonary diseases. In: Dworkin PH, ed. The national medical series for independent study: Pediatrics. New York: John Wiley & Sons, Inc., 1987:273.
3. Tachdjian MO. Orthopedic problems in childhood. In: Rudolph AM, ed. Pediatrics. 17th ed. Norwalk, Connecticut: Appleton-Century-Crofts, 1982; 1817.
4. Renshaw TS. Pediatric Orthopedics. Philadelphia: W.B. Saunders Co., 1986:66.
5. Ballard JL, Novak KK, Driver M. A simplified score for assessment of fetal maturation of newly born infants. J Pediatr 1979;95:769–774.
6. Dubowitz L. Dubowitz V, Goldberg C. Clinical assessment of gestational age in the newborn infant. J Pediatr 1970;77:1.
7. Amiel-Tison C. Neurological evaluation of the maturity of newborn infants. Arch Dis Child 1968; 43:89.
8. Farr V, Mitchell R, Neligan C, et al. The definition of some external characteristics used in the assessment of gestation age of the newborn infant. Dev Med Child Neurol 1966;8:507.

CHAPTER 3

Infant

THE INFANT HISTORY
Student Task

1. Obtain an infant history.

You are ready to begin a health maintenance visit with 2-month-old Emily Smith. If you've been reading in sequence, you know that you have a few things to do before you enter the room (remember: **preparation, observation,** and **modification**). You'll need to review: the old chart (we'll supply that information in a minute), the flow sheet for age 2 months, and the explanatory notes (these follow shortly). Remember to use this information not only to decide what questions to ask, but also to plot strategy for establishing alliances with family members and the patient. Once you begin the interview, use **observation** not only to **modify** your previously formulated plans for establishing rapport and focusing the history, but also to simultaneously begin the nontactile portion of the physical exam.

O.K., ready? Enter, introduce yourself, identify **everyone** in the room (including accompanying friends, relatives, and sibs), and ask your general opening question.

As you enter the room, you notice that little Emily is crying lustily while lying on the examining table. An older woman picks her up and attempts to soothe her by rocking her and making endearing statements to her. The baby quiets readily. She opens here eyes and smiles at the older woman. A younger woman is reading a magazine. You introduce yourself and find out that the older woman is Mrs. Kelly. The younger woman looks up briefly and tells you that she is Julie

Kates . . . You have already made important observations: Mrs. Kelly is attached to little Emily and Emily is attached to her (**attachment**). You also see that Emily is easily calmed (**temperament**) and that she has a social smile (**developmental milestone**). Of some concern to you is Ms. Kates' lack of attention to the baby's fussing (**lack of synchrony**).

What's going on here? . . . The chart notes inform you: Ms. Kates, age 16, is the natural mother. She is unmarried, lives with her own mother, and has a long history of depression. Her pregnancy was complicated by a suicide attempt. She gave the baby the natural father's last name. However, he is not involved with either her or the baby. Mrs. Kelly is the foster mother. Knowing this information before you went in to the room certainly would have helped you! It was all there, you just needed to remember to look for it. Just by saying "hello," you were able to get some information regarding affective development and psycho-social status. Your observations also confirmed at least one developmental milestone. See how much information you are able to get with your "first" infant exam before you "lay hands on."

Infant History Flow Sheets

The infant history flow sheets, along with explanatory notes, follow these comments. Familiarize yourself with their contents, although memorization isn't necessary. If you practice using them on your young patients, the most important issues will become familiar.

Table 3.1
History Flow Sheets: Infant

	History			Interval Updates	
Early Infancy Age	General Care	Growth and Development	Developmental Milestones	General Health (ROS and PMH)	Family and Psycho-Social
Two Weeks to Four Weeks	Feeding breast/ formula schedule Sleep Elimination urinary stream Hygiene navel/cir-cumcision Safety car seat crib bars/ bumpers water temp <120°	Affective Synchrony infant effect on environ-ment cueing in/mutual awareness Temperament parental perception individuality/ crying Attachment Physical State unpredictability Motor Growth	Regards face Follows to midline Reacts to sound Raises head when prone Moro + Reflex grasp + Tonic neck +	Health update Review prenatal and birth history Vitamins/ fluoride Fever control rectal thermometer Screening neonatal metabolic Vision/hearing	Review family Health and Psycho-social History Parental reaction Return to work Spousal Involvement Sibling rivalry Environment smoke detectors smoking
Two Months	Feeding breast/ formula spitting up/ solids Sleep methods used Elimination ↑ regularity Safety car seat/ potential for falls Toys age-appro-priate	Affective Synchrony fussing Temperament individuality obvious Attachment recognition of caretakers Physical State schedule ↑ regu-larity of demands Motor Growth	Smiles responsively Follows past midline Turns head and eyes to sound Raises head prone 45° Vocalizes bubbles and coos	Health update Fever control Acetaminophen Immunization contraindications Vision/hearing	Family status Child care Environment smoking

Early Infancy Explanatory Notes (Two Weeks through Four Months)

GENERAL CARE

Feeding

Is the baby nursed, bottled, or both? If nursing, how often? Both breasts offered at each feeding? How long on each side? Has the mother experienced any breast infections or significant nipple soreness? How have these been dealt with? If bottle feeding, what formula is used? Is it iron fortified? How many ounces does the baby take per feeding? How often is he fed?

Table 3.1—*continued*

	History			Interval Updates	
Early Infancy Age	General Care	Growth and Development	Developmental Milestones	General Health (ROS and PMH)	Family and Psycho-Social
	Feeding breast/ formula solids/cup # meals	Affective Temperament ↑ stability Attachment main agenda	Shows excitement upon recognition of familiar people Follows 180°	Health update Immunization reaction contraindications	Family status
Four Months	Sleep own room Safety gates/playpen walker Toys age-appropriate	Physical Motor new skills Growth	Smiles, laughs, gurgles Prone head high raises body with hands Rolls front to back Sits with support head steady Holds rattle briefly TNR − MORO ±	Teething drooling Habits self-soothing Vision/hearing	
Later Infancy Age	Feeding breast/ formula solids/cup # meals	Affective Temperament highly visible predictable	Squeals/ Raspberries Sits alone ± Some weight bearing Rolls F to B/ B to F	Health update Vitamins/ fluoride iron fortified cereal Fever control Acetaminophen	Family status
	Sleep bottle in bed resistance	Attachment stranger/ separation anxiety	No head lag Reaches Transfers ± Turns to sound	Immunization reaction contraindications	
Six Months	Safety car seat high chair w/ harness covered wall sockets supervised bath Toys favorite parental interaction	Autonomy/ Independence struggle between dependence/ independence Physical Motor mobility/ autonomy Growth		Teething Habits Vision/hearing	

Table 3.1—*continued*

	History			Interval Updates	
Later Infancy Age	General Care	Growth and Development	Developmental Milestones	General Health (ROS and PMH)	Family and Psycho-Social
Nine Months	Feeding weaning/ # meals finger and table foods appetite decrease salt usage Sleep night crying Safety car seat/open windows stairwells/ gates/cords walkers avoidance of unsafe foods and toys	Affective Temperament predictable responses Attachment clinging Autonomy/ independence main agenda/ struggles autonomy encouraged freedom to explore and to be messy Cognitive objective permanence causality Physical Motor autonomy Growth basic dietary needs	MaMa/DaDa nonspecific Sits alone Pulls to stand Creeps Transfers well Feeds self finger foods Peek-a-boo Parachute reflex +	Health update Immunization reaction contraindications Poison control ipecac poison control # Vision/hearing	Family status
Twelve Months	Feeding whole milk table foods Sleep night crying Safety car seat, sharp objects, household poisons Dental care cleaning by parents	Affective Temperament parental assessment Attachment clinging Autonomy/ independence temper tantrums Physical Motor exploration	MaMa/DaDa specific Other meaningful words ± Cruises Walks with support Pincer grasp Bang two blocks together Social games pat-a-cake, so-big waves bye-bye Looks for hidden objects (Formal DDST alternative)	Health update Immunization reaction contraindications Screening anemia Habits Poison control ipecac poison control # Vision/hearing	Family status

Are there problems with feeding (e.g., spitting up)? Does the baby seem satisifed? As the baby gets older is there increasing regularity to his demands (e.g., Is there a schedule?)? Have solids been introduced? If so, what kinds? How much? How often? Any affect noticeable on baby (e.g., gassy, happy)? Have liquids been offered by cup? If so, what kinds?

Sleeping

What is the baby's sleep pattern like (e.g., how long does he sleep at one time and how often does he fall asleep?)? What method is used to put the baby down to sleep (e.g., is he put down immediately after a feeding? Is he rocked to sleep or is he put in his crib awake?)? Where does baby sleep (e.g., in a cradle, mother's bed, or own crib? . . . own room?)? Is schedule being established as he gets older? Does he sleep through the night?

Elimination

How often does baby have a bowel movement? What is consistency? As baby gets older, is there increasing regularity to his pattern? How many wet diapers (approximately) does baby produce in a 24-hour period? For boys, is stream powerful and straight?

Hygiene

How often is baby bathed? Where is he bathed? What soap and shampoo are used? How are the navel and circumcision sites cared for?

Safety

Is a car seat being used? What type? Where is it located in car? (e.g., front or back seat, facing front or back windows?) Ask a general question to introduce the topic of household safety, such as, have you made any changes in the household yet to protect the baby from injury? Has water temperature in the home been turned down to <120°? How close together are crib slats? Are there bumpers in the crib? Is a play pen

used? If so, for what purposes? Is baby left on a bed or changing table while unattended? As the infant approaches 4–6 months, ask, are stairway gates being installed (as baby begins to move around)? Is a walker used?

Toys

What toys are being used?

GROWTH AND DEVELOPMENT

During the first weeks and months of their infant's life, parents experience dramatic changes in their own lives. Developmental history-taking affords the clinician an opportunity to inquire about baby's progress while simultaneously inquiring about parents' progress. For example, when discussing synchrony, you are interested in finding out what effect the infant has had on the environment, as well as whether or not parents are able to "cue-in" to baby's signals. In other words, when you ask how much fussing or crying the baby does, also ask how parents interpret and intervene when baby cries. Similarly, when discussing motor development, ask about the baby's latest "accomplishments" while also inquiring about whether or not these meet parental expectations.

Affective Development

Synchrony.   Do parents express uncertainty in deciding what baby's demands mean? As baby gets older (2–4 months), do they find it easier to figure out what baby wants? Does baby have predictable fussy periods? When are these and how long do they last?

Temperament.   Ask parents what this baby is like. How much of the time does he seem content or fussy? Does he seem to be a happy baby? As he gets older, do the parents perceive certain personality traits?

Attachment.   Is infant beginning to show preferential response to parents voice? As baby gets older, does he show visual recognition of main caretakers and is he beginning to respond with pleasure or excitement towards them?

Physical Development

State. The very young infant is predictably unpredictable in his sleep-wake cycles and feeding patterns. As he grows, the regularity of his demands and periods of alertness increase. What is this infant like?

Motor. How active is the baby? What are his motor accomplishments? Do parents feel his body is getting stronger?

Growth. Do parents feel he is growing adequately?

DEVELOPMENTAL MILESTONES

Ask parents: What is he doing? Does he make sounds other than crying? Does he react in any way to sound or visual signals? What is he doing with his body? These are general ways to get at the information being sought in this category. That way, if there is something that the baby is not yet doing, you will not worry the parent if you ask the question in a more general manner. At some point, also find out if there is anything that the baby could once do and is now no longer doing (this is called "loss of milestones"). You will need to confirm this information during your physical exam.

Does the 2–4-week-old regard a human face and follow 90° to either side from the midline? Does he display a physical reaction to a loud sound? Does he raise his head slightly off the bed when placed on his belly? Does he still have a moro and a reflex grasp? He will acquire a tonic neck reflex by about age one month (read about this is in the physical exam).

Does the 2-month-old smile when he sees a human face? Does he follow an object beyond 90° (past the midline)? Does he turn his head and eyes towards the source of a loud sound? Does he raise his head to at least a 45° angle from a prone position? Does he make bubbling or cooing noises?

Does the 4-month-old show excitement when he encounters people he knows? Does he follow an object around a 180° arc (from one side across the midline to the other side)? Does he smile, laugh, gurgle, or squeal? When he is prone, does he hold his head high and raise his body off the table with his arms? Is he beginning to roll from front to back? Is his head steady when he is supported in a sitting position? Does he briefly hold a rattle when it is placed in his hand? (This is different from the reflex grasp of a newborn). He will no longer have a tonic neck reflex. A moro may still be present up to six months.

GENERAL HEALTH

Does the baby seem healthy? At a first encounter, review the prenatal and birth history. Obtain an interval update on review of systems and past medical history. For a healthy infant, the **General Care** section covers most of these topics.

Vitamins/fluoride

Are fluoride supplements or vitamins being used? Where does family live? (Water system fluoride content varies from town to town.)

Fever Control

Do parents own and know how to use a rectal thermometer? Is there infant acetaminophen in the house? Do parents understand when to administer it and what the dosage should be? Has the baby received it? If so, why?

Screening

Did baby have neonatal metabolic screen performed (i.e., for congenital hypothyroidism)?

Immunizations

When immunizations are scheduled review patient and household contraindications. This includes reviewing reactions to prior immunizations.

Teething

Is the baby drooling or teething?

Habits

Does the baby suck his thumb or display any other self-soothing behavior?

Vision/Hearing

Does the baby seem to see and hear?

FAMILY/PSYCHOSOCIAL

At a first visit obtain a family medical and psychosocial history. This may include drawing a family tree. At each subsequent visit briefly ask how everyone in the family is doing. This may include reviewing the family tree.

There are many questions you may pose at this point. **Modify** them according to each individual family. Ask about the adjustment to life with the new baby. Have there been any major family medical problems since the baby was last seen? Has anything else happened at home (changes or crises)? How are siblings doing? What are childcare arrangements and how are they working? Is mother planning to return to work outside the home? How involved is the other parent and is he (or she) a source of emotional and financial support? Are parents married? Who lives in the household? Are there other sources of financial and emotional support? Is babysitting (for parental leisure time) available? Have parents begun to take advantage of it?

Environment: Does anyone in the household smoke? Are there smoke detectors?

Later Infancy Explanatory Notes (Six Months through Twelve Months)

GENERAL CARE

Feeding

Continue to ask breast/bottle questions. Does the baby drink any other milk beside formula or breast? Does baby eat solids? If so, what kinds in what amounts? How many meals per day? Is a cup used? If so, for what?

Are finger or table foods offered? Which ones? How does baby handle them? Are foods salted? As the baby approaches age 1, does he show decreasing appetite and/or a resistance to being fed from a spoon? Does the baby take a bottle to bed? If so, what liquid is in bottle?

Sleep

Does the baby show resistance to going to sleep? Is there nighttime crying? How are these issues handled by parents?

Safety

Ask a general question: Have you made any changes in the household yet to protect the baby from injury? If so, what have you done? Specific questions may include use of the following preventive measures: car seat, safety strap on high chair, covers on wall socket, gates on stairways, protection from open windows, locked storage of medicines and cleaning agents, childproof locks on drawers or cabinets with sharp objects. Are foods and toys that may be aspirated avoided (e.g., nuts, hot dogs, popcorn, small toys)? Is a walker used?

Toys

What toys does baby prefer? Does he have a favorite?

Dental

Do parents clean infant's teeth (with a gauze or wash cloth)?

GROWTH AND DEVELOPMENT

During the second half of the first year, the infant's behavior and personality become more obvious and predictable to caretakers. During this period, many babies develop stranger and separation anxiety. This may be manifested by the infant who now "hangs on" to familiar people and situations. As the end of the first year approaches (as the child is fully immersed in the process of separation and individuation), struggles between baby and parents erupt. In the process of achieving autonomy, the baby becomes involved in an unconscious struggle between his need for dependence and his desire for independence. As his motor abilities increase, his ability to be physically autonomous increases also. He becomes "too busy" to eat and resists being fed. The growth rate slows dramatically.

Affective Development

Temperament. What is the baby's personality like? Are his reactions increasingly predictable?

Attachment. How does the baby react when you leave him? How does the baby react to strangers?

Autonomy/Independence. Is the baby showing some signs of independence? What are they (e.g., wanting to feed himself, resisting diaper changes)? Is he allowed to explore the house? Where can he go? Does he make a mess at the table? How does he react when you say no? Does he have temper tantrums? How do you handle these issues?

Cognitive Development

Does the 9–12-month-old show interest in finding objects that are hidden in his presence (object permanence)? Does he show interest in wind up toys (causality)?

Physical Development

Motor. What are his new skills? Is he exploring? Are you satisfied with his progress?

Growth. Are you worried about his growth or appetite?

DEVELOPMENTAL MILESTONES

Does the six-month-old squeal or "make raspberries" (make sounds by pushing air out through pursed lips)? Does he sit alone (about half of six-month-olds can do this)? Does he bear some weight when held in a standing position? Does he roll from front to back and back to front? When he is pulled from the supine position (by holding onto his hands), does his head lag behind his body (it shouldn't)? Does he reach for objects placed in front of him? Does he transfer objects from one hand to another (most can do this by 7 months)? Does he turn his body towards the source of a noise?

Does the nine-month-old babble Dada/Mama nonspecifically? Does he sit alone? Does he pull himself up in the crib? Does he creep? Does he transfer objects well? Does he feed himself finger foods? Does he like to play peek-a-boo?

Does the twelve-month-old say mama or dada in the correct context? Does he have any other words that have a meaning to you? Does he walk around holding on (cruise)? Does he take steps yet? Does he pick up small objects using his thumb and forefinger (pincer grasp) rather than using his whole fist? Does he bang objects together? Does he like to play games such as peek-a-boo, pat-a-cake, or so-big? Does he look for hidden objects? Some pediatricians choose to perform a formal developmental screening test at this time (e.g., Denver II-see Appendix).

GENERAL HEALTH

Obtain an interval update.

Vitamins/Fluoride

Review vitamin and fluoride use. Is cereal iron fortified?

Fever Control

Review acetaminophen and thermometer availability and usage.

Screening

Many pediatricians screen for anemia during the second half of the infant's first year. Has the baby been screened?

Immunizations

When immunizations are scheduled, review patient and household contraindications. This includes reviewing reactions to prior immunizations.

Teething

Does he have any teeth yet? How many does he have? How is baby handling teething? What remedies have been used?

Habits

Does the baby suck his thumb, or display any other self-soothing behavior (e.g., head banging)?

Poison control

Is poison control phone number posted at home? Is ipecac available? Do parents understand procedure for use?

Vision/Hearing

Does the baby seem to see and hear well?

FAMILY/PSYCHOSOCIAL

Obtain an interval update. Any problems? How is everyone doing? Are parents enjoying the baby? What are the child care arrangements?

There are many areas you may explore. Review those listed in Early Infancy Explanatory Notes on Family/Psycho-Social. **Modify** your line of questioning based on your existing data base and your **observations.**

THE PHYSICAL EXAM OF THE INFANT

Student Task

1. Examine an infant.

General Approach

You now have quite a bit of information about your young patient and his or her family. Your physical exam is also partially done because you remembered to **observe** as you were speaking to them. Continue this process as you prepare to "lay hands on."

❓ **After obtaining history and making initial observations, what else must you do before you proceed further? . . . I will remind you again and again (because it's a common error made by beginners) . . . Wash your hands!!**

Let's get back to the exam. Here's an example: The four-month-old is a smiley cooperative child. She's awake for many more hours than the newborn (**state**). Her personality has become more defined (**temperament**). Her mom has just told you that she loves being in the center of the action where there are sights and sounds to distract her. When she's been fed, burped, and changed, she's content to spend time in her infant seat just "taking it all in." She's a great socializer. She turns to her mother and father's voice and greets them with great smiles which mom assures you are meant just for them (**attachment**). Whenever she's placed belly-down in her crib, she immediately loves to practice rolling over onto her back (**motor development**).

While you're talking with mom, watch the baby. Study her **general facial** and **body appearance.** How alert is she? Does she smile at mom? Does she follow her mom with her gaze? Does she react to sudden noises? Is their interaction loving and affectionate? If she's placed on the examining table, does she attempt to roll over? (Make sure someone is always at her side to prevent her from falling!) Is there something unusual about her facial or body appearance?

Once you're comfortable with the technical aspects, you will find the exams on young infants, during the first 6 months, less stressful than exams on older infants and toddlers.

Smile at the baby. She'll smile back. Her friendliness will continue for the majority of your encounter. Until the baby is 6–9 months old, you will not need to use any special tricks to defer fears (there aren't any). As long as you smile, and your voice and touch are gentle and friendly, she'll allow you to proceed. Make sure your hands and stethescope are warm (this is true for any age). Let her mom place her on the examining table and have her stay nearby while you do the exam. Start your exam at her head and proceed in a downward fashion. But wait. She will resist and cry when you make her uncomfortable. Defer the difficult parts of the exam until the end (ears, mouth and hips).

The real test begins with your six- to nine-month-old patient. Remember Carl Davos? Carl, at nine months was in the midst of working through stranger and separation anxiety. You were able to minimize those predictable fears by altering your body language, and giving him time to familiarize himself with you and your instruments. You distracted him by allowing him to do what he enjoyed most: handling things and putting things into his mouth. At this age, it may still be possible for you to examine him on the examining table, as long as mommy or daddy stay nearby (the uniqueness of a child's development and temperament will influence this). Allow him (and watch while he does it) to transfer small objects (the rubber bulb on your otoscope is always handy) as you begin your exam. At some point in the latter half of the first year, he may resist lying down. Do the obvious: If he resists lying down, defer that until the end.[1,2]

By now I'm sure you've noticed that the order of "head to toe" will become more and more jumbled as resistance of your patient increases. That's o.k., as long as you remember to add the missing details at the end. At this age, children begin to enjoy practicing some of their motor accomplishments. They won't mind being moved around a bit, once they've gotten to know you. So, pulling them to sit or stand, to complete your exam will probably be fun for them.

The infant approaching age one has begun to take another developmental leap.

❓ **What are the major developmental milestones around age one? (Check your history flow sheet.) That's right. The infant is developing increasing motor skills. He may be taking a few careful steps. If he hasn't done that yet, he will be cruising briskly! One way to make a child at this age feel less intimidated, is to allow him to "cruise" around while you are taking the history. Don't forget to observe his gait.**

By age one, your patient may be **very** clingy. The examining table will be the **enemy.** Gradually draw your chair closer during the interview so he has time to get used to you. It will now be necessary for you to sit (vs. stand) while you examine him.

Modification of body language (eyes, voice, and stance) with a gradual transition from ignoring to direct contact becomes crucial to your success. Most of the exam can be done while he sits in his parent's lap. Begin with a game: ("pat-a-cake" or "soo big"); begin with the extremities (count fingers or toes), and begin touching with a gradual "to and fro" motion (rather than constant). **Modify** the order as you need to. Don't hesitate to stop when you need to. Use words that are familiar and concrete (momma, dada, cookie). You will need to be a creative master of distraction.[1,2]

Keep the details of the newborn exam in mind. Continue to look for congenital anomalies. Even though the instructions will not be duplicated below, the maneuvers still apply in the infant exam. What will be highlighted from now on are the areas most likely to have significance for the age group being discussed.

As a final note, continue to **observe** parent-child interaction (both verbal and physical) throughout the encounter. This text emphasizes the initial parts of the clinical process (the history and physical). Once you have mastered these, you will be ready to work on the interpretative (or latter) aspects of the process. At that time, you will be required to assess how well (or poorly) your patient is functioning. The contribution of family relationships to a child's wellbeing cannot be overestimated. The clinical encounter provides a golden opportunity to observe these relationships.

Measurements

Having been weighed and measured by the nurse, the baby is probably stripped down to his diaper. If not, then have his mom do it. If you haven't yet plotted length and weight on the growth charts, do it now (plot head circumference too if this has been measured). Prematures (especially those born months early) may need to be plotted according to their gestational age, rather than their chronologic age. This method of plotting adjusted age is most commonly used during the first year of life when the premature's growth is still "catching up" to that of a baby born at term. **Plotting measurements on growth curves during the encounter, rather than afterwards,** allows you to perform a more focused and rational history and physical.

Review the developmental columns in your history section. As you proceed, you will be able to confirm milestones. The developmental achievements may need to be "adjusted" downward (for prematures) in the same fashion as their growth parameters.

With the wary infant, your **games** can include assessing development. In fact, you may reverse the entire order of the exam and begin with the neuro-developmental assessment. Thinking about general appearance (state of consciousness, mood, activity level, brightness of gaze) should always come first. Then zero in on specifics. For simplicity, we'll begin here in the traditional fashion.

Skin

Observe color and turgor. Note and describe rashes and birthmarks (e.g., nevi, hemangiomas, depigmented and cafe au lait spots).

Strawberry hemangiomas grow rapidly during infancy. No intervention is necessary unless a vital structure is threatened by encroachment (i.e., eye, larynx). The appearance of these vascular tumors is a major concern for parents. Their usual reaction is: "He didn't have this when he was born." Reassure them that this type of hemangioma is often invisible at birth. It will continue to grow rapidly in size and palpability during the first 6 to 12 months and then begin to involute. Almost all "strawberries" have resolved completely by middle childhood.

❓ Which hemangiomas do not involute? . . . Right! Port Wine stains.

The infant under one month may be jaundiced. Note the presence of jaundice and the distribution. This is most common in breast fed infants. Breast feeding jaundice gradually resolves by age 4 to 6 weeks. After the second week of life, worsening jaundice is usually of pathologic significance.

Once the baby begins solid foods (usually four to six months), a generous intake of orange and yellow fruits and vegetables may give the skin an orange hue (**carotenemia**) which is particularly accentuated on the palms and soles. This is sometimes confused with jaundice. Carotenemia never involves the conjunctivae. The temporal link to food intake should be established.

The following are common rashes which appear during the first few months of life. You will see these when you examine both well and sick infants. Rashes which principally involve the diaper area will be discussed when we take the diaper off.

Infantile acne: This appears on the face of an infant during the first few months of life and lasts several months. It resembles adolescent acne and consists of papules and pustules with surrounding erythema. Its presence is not predictive of teenage acne.

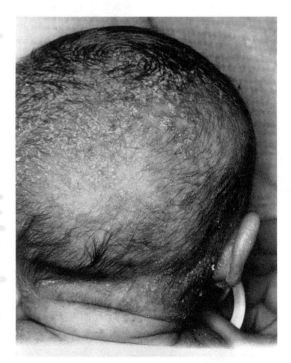

Figure 3.1. Cradle cap. Reproduced with permission. Hurwitz S. Clinical pediatric dermatology. Philadelphia: W.B. Saunders, 1981:13. Photo courtesy of Sidney Hurwitz, M.D.

Seborrhea (Figure 3.1): This appears during the first few months of life and is usually self-resolving after several months. The greasy, yellow tinged, scaly rash involving the scalp is called cradle cap. The face and eyebrows may also be involved. The skin behind the ears and/or the folds of the neck, axilla, groin, and umbilicus take on a reddened, scaly appearance. It is not pruritic.

Infantile atopic dermatitis (Figure 3.2) (**eczema**): This begins slightly later than seborrhea (age two to six months). The skin is dry. The rash is red and may be crusted or vesiculated. It is intensely pruritic. Excoriations are common. It involves the face (especially the cheeks), occasionally the scalp, and the extremities in a symmetrical distribution on the extensor surfaces. The infantile form and distribution of atopic dermatitis may last for several years. In many cases, there is a strong family history of atopy.

These newborn rashes may affect the young infant, too:

Erythema toxicum: This is sometimes still present at two weeks of age. Rarely, it first appears at 10 to 14 days.

Miliaria: These lesions may be asymptomatic, clear tiny vesicles without an erythematous base (*m. crystallina*). As the eruption intensifies, they become pruritic and papulovesicular with an erythematous halo base (*m. rubra*, prickly heat). They are found anywhere on the body but are worse in clothed areas of the body.

Transient Neonatal Pustular Melanosis: The macules that appear after the rupture of the vesicles and pustules may remain up to two to three months.

Intertrigo: This is a nonspecific skin fold irritation. The axilla, neck and groin folds become red and may denude the superficial skin layer. This produces weeping fluid. The macerated skin may become secondarily infected.

Herpes simplex: The devastating herpes of the newborn may not present until week two of life. Grouped vesicles on an erythematous base should alert you to consider this diagnosis in the very young infant.

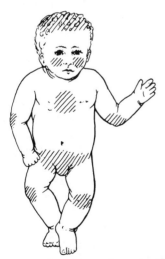

Figure 3.2. Distribution of atopic dermatitis during infancy: cheeks, trunk, extremities (extensor surfaces). Reproduced with permission. Fleisher GR, Ludwig S. eds. Textbook of pediatric emergency medicine. 2nd ed. Baltimore: Williams & Wilkins, 1988;773.

Head

Measure the head circumference. Assess the head shape for asymmetries and unusual contours (molding resolves in the first weeks to month). Feel the head, suture lines and measure the fontanelle sizes.

The head size and rate of growth (in part) reflect the growth of the underlying brain. It is necessary to follow head growth during the first year (or longer—if there are suspicions of an abnormality) of life, because half of ultimate brain growth is completed by age nine months and 75% is completed by age 2.[3]

Shape: A markedly assymetric head may be the result of premature fusion of the cranial sutures (called **craniosynostosis**). This becomes more pronounced as the head grows. This also will produce ridging of the involved suture lines and sometimes a head that grows too slowly.

The **head shape of a premature** (particularly those born 2 to 3 months early) is characteristically **long and narrow** (in a longitudinal direction) with the sides flattened. The tiny premie, by himself, is unable to life his head up (remember we spoke earlier about adjusting "developmental milestones" downward like growth parameters?). In addition, his skull is softer and more malleable than that of a full-term infant. Consequently, he will spend most of his first few months of life lying with his moldable skull turned to one side or another. This flattening effect becomes less noticeable when the head is covered by hair.

Another common variation in contour is a **flattened occiput.** This is particularly seen during the first half of the first year in infants who spend a lot of time lying on their back. This is accentuated in babies whose development is slow and who are lacking in strong muscle tone.

As you feel along the skull of the infant, you may notice some hardened prominences from resolving cephalohematomas. These slowly resolve over many months.

Sutures and Fontanelles: Ridging (or overriding) of sutures should resolve by age six months. There is gradual progressive fusion of the suture lines and, therefore, closure of the fontanelles. Although there are other fontanelles which are sometimes palpable at birth, the two whose progress is most important to follow are: the anterior and posterior fontanelles. The posterior fontanelle should be closed by approximately age two months. The anterior fontanelle closes between 6 to 18 months (age 2 by the latest). In some normal infants, it may close as early as 4 to 5 months. If there is doubt as to whether it is normal size (e.g., too big or too small), there are reference tables for normals. Like all other developmental processes, this is a gradual progression. You must assess fontanelle size in the context of head size, shape, and the general wellbeing of the child.

Check to see that the anterior fontanelle doesn't bulge.

❓ **Can you adequately assess whether the anterior fontanelle is bulging (or sunken)** **while the baby is recumbent? No! He must be upright (to eliminate the effects of gravity). If it still bulges when he's upright, what does that possibly indicate?: increased intracranial pressure (e.g., as you might see in a child with meningitis). By the way, if the fontanelle is very sunken, the baby may be dehydrated.**

If there are visible pulsations, take the pulse that way. Percussion of the head in children with open fontanelles doesn't yield useful information.

Auscultation of the head isn't a part of a routine exam in childhood. Cranial bruits up to age 5 are too common in normal children to have pathologic significance if found in the context of a normal exam; they may also signify anemia or vascular malformations (there are more reliable signs of anemia).

Hair

The quantity, texture, and pattern of hair should be noted. Newborn hair is often totally lost by the first few months of age. Replacement may take many months.

The flattened occiput of the infant who spends a good deal of time on his back will also have thinned-out hair. There may even be a bald spot.

Face

You've looked for striking abnormalities in general facial or body appearance. As you begin to zero in on specifics, look again at the whole face for asymmetries, lesions, etc. Is she bright and alert, calm, wary, or sleeping? Or does she have a dull, pale, and disinterested appearance? Observations such as these may point towards hidden problems. For instance, the infant with untreated **congenital hypothyroidism** is inactive and coarse-featured. Her skin is dry, and her hair is dull and dry. As myxedema involves her face, she develops puffy eyelids, and the appearance of small, widely spaced eyes with a depressed nasal bridge. Her mouth is open, and her thickened tongue protrudes; her cry is hoarse; her neck is thick and short.

You can observe all of this without even undressing her! When you do, you will find that her skin is cool and mottled and she is hypotonic; her abdomen is distended and she is likely to have an umbilical hernia.

Eyes

Assess shape, size, and symmetry (start by examining the whole eye, then focus in on the individual structures: sclera, iris, pupil, conjunctiva, and lids). Note pupillary size, equality, reaction to light, and accommodation. Iris color change (to brown or green) may not be complete until one year of age. Evert the lower lids slightly to check for the absence of pallor.

Obviously, performing a thorough assessment of the eyes requires that they be open. The less you have to pry the eyes open and battle to keep them open, the easier your exam will be. We've already mentioned that lifting the newborn upright and moving him about will aid you. During the first few months of life (if you catch the baby with his eyes open), he should not object too strenuously to your shining light. An older infant isn't usually as compliant. To get him to open his eyes, you may want to stand behind the mother as she holds him upright over her shoulder (as if she were burping him). To get him to keep the eyes open, hold up an attractive object in one hand (for the baby to fix on) while you hold your ophthalmoscope in the other hand. Another trick is to offer the baby something to suck on (he'll concentrate on that).

Tears may not be produced in volume until 2 to 4 months of age. A congenitally obstructed nasolacrimal (tear) duct becomes symptomatic within the first few weeks of life (as the normal drainage path for eye secretions is blocked). The parent will note that one or both eyes tear and/or retain mucoid, crusted, or even purulent material. The conjunctivae are usually only slightly reddened. Run you finger downward starting just above the inner canthus, along the side of the nose. This will frequently produce a diagnostic "pop" of retained secretions from the nasolacrimal sac proximal to the obstruction. If the eyes are very injected and/or produce large amounts of purulent material, then the diagnosis is more likely infectious conjunctivitis.

To test for visual acuity, have him fix on your light or on the brightly colored (or boldly patterned) object (or your face). Have him follow in all directions of gaze. When he is old enough to reach out, offer him something to reach for. These are reasonable tests for visual acuity during infancy.

Shine your light on his face. The corneal reflection of the light should be symmetric in both eyes. If the corneal reflection is unequal, or range of motion of either eye is incomplete, or the eyes don't always move together, suspect **strabismus.** In addition, if the child objects (particularly on one side more than the other) to having his line of vision interfered with, suspect strabismus. **Pseudostrabismus** (or the appearance of strabismus without dysfunction) is seen in some children with epicanthal folds. In these children, the corneal light reflection will be symmetric and the eyes will move together.

Children with eye misalignment or other visual problems (e.g., unequal refractive errors) that result in unequal retinal images are at risk for amblyopia. "**Amblyopia** is a unilateral or bilateral reduction in visual acuity (in the absence of any visual organic lesion), despite appropriate optical correction" (e.g., correction of refractive errors).[4] Amblyopia is often preventable with early diagnosis and treatment of the underlying cause.

The **alternate cover test** is one type of strabismus screen that may uncover a subtle strabismus. This test assumes that each eye has central vision. During the alternate cover test, you need an object that the child will fixate on (e.g., a toy or other attractive object) and you need something to cover the patient's eye without touching it. Some examiners prefer to use their thumb for the occluder which is then moved from eye to eye like a swinging pendulum (the rest of the hand acts as the fulcrum). You may also

Figure 3.3. Alternate cover test: once the child is fixating, shift the occluder repeatedly from eye to eye while observing the recently uncovered eye for any movement. If movement is observed, suspect strabismus.

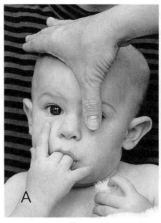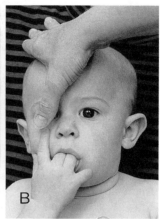

require an assistant to hold up the interesting object at some distance from the child if the parent is occupied by holding the infant. The test is performed like this:

The interesting object is held up for the child to fixate on. Once the child is fixating, cover one eye in an unobtrusive manner. After several seconds, shift the cover to the opposite eye (allowing no time in between for binocular vision). Observe the recently uncovered eye as it assumes fixation for any movement. You can repeatedly shift the cover from eye to eye, always observing the eye being uncovered for any movement. If there is movement observed, suspect strabismus.

Practice looking at the retina. You have been instructed to examine the adult patient's right eye with your right eye and vice versa. If your patient is too young to actively cooperate, try a switch from the traditional method: use your right eye to examine the patient's left eye and vice versa. This means that you will be coming across the patient's face during your exam. To distract him from looking directly at the light, hold up a toy between you and the patient (one hand on the ophthalmoscope, one hand on the toy). The baby will gaze in your direction, but rather than looking directly at you he will look at the toy. (If this is too awkward for you, perform the exam in the traditional manner). In either case, focus first on the orange-colored retina and vessels. Search for

hemorrhages, exudates, or abnormal pigmentation. These appear as spots and patches on the retina. Locate the disc and look for sharp disc margins. Follow this by looking for the macula which is temporal to the disc. In certain diseases, the macula becomes pigmented or fragmented. Admittedly, this exam is much easier to talk about than to actually perform on a "moving target." Take it slowly and don't expect to see all of these areas the first time you attempt it. Even the most experienced pediatrician has difficulty with this exam.

Ears

Inspect the ears. Note any drainage from the canal. Confirm that he can hear by making a loud noise behind him to see if he reacts to the sound. If he is too young to turn his head very far, hold a bell off to each side and see if he turns his eyes or head in reaction. If that doesn't work, slam a door and see if he startles. Admittedly, this is "gross" and somewhat subjective; but without very sophisticated apparatus, it's the best you can do in the office with a very young infant. Defer otoscopic exam till the end of the physical.

Parental concerns about their infant's vision or hearing should be taken very seriously. Their subjective impressions about either, particularly in infancy, are very accurate.

Nose

Check for drainage and patency (describe color and thickness if drainage is present). healthy mucosa is pink. Upper respiratory infections (frequent during infancy) are accompanied by reddened nasal mucosa. Listen for congestion or snorting. A wide otoscope head will allow you to see in the lower half of the nose. You will see the lower turbinates and parts of the middle ones.

Mouth

Inspect lips, gums, anterior tongue, and teeth. You may use a tongue depressor for this. Many young infants have **thrush.** This is a candidal infection manifested by white plaques on the tongue and/or buccal mucosa. This may be associated with a diaper rash. To differentiate this from retained milk (which this resembles) try to gently scrape a plaque off. Thrush does not scrape off easily and may bleed when this maneuver is attempted.

The timing of tooth eruption is somewhat variable. The order of eruption is less so. The first teeth to appear are usually the lower central incisors (one at a time at 6–8 mos.), followed shortly thereafter by the upper incisors (8–9 mos.). The lower and upper lateral incisors erupt during the latter part of the first year. A one-year-old may also have begun eruption of lower and upper first molars. Less often the teeth do not begin to erupt until age one. Further delayed eruption is unusual and may be associated with some disorders of the pituitary axis, rickets, or some syndromes. Note any unusual shape or coloring of teeth. Some abnormalities include: iron preparations stain the teeth brown; prenatal tetracycline exposure stains teeth yellow; dentin and enamel dysplasias may exhibit yellow to brownish teeth; and, excessive fluoride ingestion may cause the teeth to have chalky white spots. Children with one of the ectodermal dysplasia syndromes may have pointed "tepee"-shaped teeth.

Several months prior to the first eruption at approximately ages 3–4 mos., the baby begins to drool and mouth or bite available objects. Don't force the mouth open at this point in the exam. If you need to do this, defer it until the end of the exam. Note sounds or words the baby utters.

Neck

Inspect for bulges (e.g., cysts) and thyroid enlargement. In order to **really** inspect the thyroid of an infant, the neck should be hyperextended; if you don't do this, you will miss many goiters. Palpate for adenopathy. **A few small mobile anterior or posterior cervical nodes are found in most healthy children** (high up in the triangles). If he's supine, pull him to sitting while holding his hands and observe his head control both during this maneuver and when he's sitting up.

Check range of motion and observe for torticollis.

❓ **What is torticollis? As we mentioned in the previous chapter, torticollis is a lateral head tilt with chin rotated to the opposite side. This is difficult to diagnose in the newborn. It becomes obvious in the first few weeks after birth.**

In the child with torticollis extend the neck and palpate for a hard "mass" (contracted, fibrosed muscle) within the sternocleido-mastoid muscle on the involved side. This gradually enlarges to a maximum at age 5–6 weeks and may be as large as an inch long. It gradually regresses over the next several

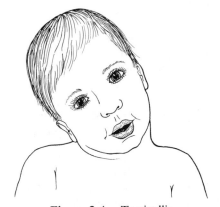

Figure 3.4. Torticollis.

months and may take as long as a half year. Therapy consists of muscle stretching exercises.

Until the latter part of the first year, nuchal rigidity is not a reliable sign of meningeal irritation. You will learn to evaluate neck "suppleness" in the next chapter.

Thorax and Upper Extremities

Inspect clavicles, thorax, and upper extremities. Observe for spontaneous symmetric movements. Check the arms for range of motion, strength, bulk, and tone. Examine hands and fingers. If the infant is old enough to reach out and grab objects, present an interesting object just outside her range. Move it all around her until you have satisfied yourself that her upper extremity range of motion is normal and full. (Then allow her to hold whatever you had tempted her with). Feel along the lengths of the clavicles. Palpate the supraclavicular areas and axillae for lymph nodes or masses. Supraclavicular adenopathy isn't normal and if found may reflect lymph gland disease or intrathoracic pathology. A few small axillary lymph nodes without significant adenopathy in other areas may be found in healthy children. The sternum should be examined for pectus excavatum or carinatum. Examine the breasts.

❓ **A milky discharge is seen from the nipple of a two-week-old male infant. Mom is concerned. What should you tell her? Tell her about physiologic galactorrhea.**

Cardiorespiratory

Inspect and palpate the precordium. A convenient time to remember to palpate pulses is during your cardiac exam. Alternatively, palpate pulses during the extremity exam. Palpate the brachial pulses simultaneously; palpate the right brachial and femoral pulse simultaneously. The femoral pulse should not be delayed.

❓ **Weak or absent femoral pulses should make you wonder about what cardiac lesion? Yes! Coarctation of the aorta.**

You should already have looked for cyanosis.

The PMI in infancy is felt in the 4th intercostal space just to the left of the midclavicular line. If you do not find it there, try to ascertain if it is in an abnormal location. The PMI is difficult to palpate in babies; its location may be helpful if you feel it is clearly abnormal. The abnormal location may reflect cardiac enlargement, cardiac malposition, or lung disease. Thrills and heaves also reflect cardiac pathology.

An alternative approach here is to auscultate first if the baby is calm or sleeping. In this age group, especially when you do not suspect heart or lung disease, auscultation of the heart is much more important than palpation of the PMI. That doesn't mean you shouldn't perform both maneuvers. It just means that if you are dealing with an older infant who is likely to resist you, auscultate when you have the opportunity.

Auscultate the heart over the precordium, axillae, neck, and back using both the bell and the diaphragm. You should listen with the infant lying down and sitting up. This may require some extra distraction techniques. The younger infant quiets with the pacifier or while being fed. For the recumbent exam, the older infant does best while being cradled by a parent. The parent will help to soothe his child while you listen. For distraction, you can also hold up something for the child to look at, or hand him something to hold.

Auscultate for rate and rhythm.

❓ **The heart rate may vary with what? Yes, respiration (sinus arrythmia). This is actually an electrocardiographic diagnosis. However, it is so common (particularly as children get older), that in the absence of signs or symptoms of cardiac disease, pediatricians make this diagnosis clinically.**

Next, concentrate on each heart sound individually. S1 is loudest over the apex, and S2 is loudest at the upper left sternal border. S2 splitting and the normal widening with inspiration should be noted. A normal S3 may be heard at the lower left sternal border or apex. The differential diagnosis of abnormal heart sounds is beyond the scope of this text. At this point your main goals in listening to them should be to learn to identify them individually and to appreciate what "normal" intensity, quality, and variation sound like.

After you have listened to the heart sounds, listen in between them for a murmur. Identify whether or not it is in systole, diastole, or both (and if you can, decide how much of each phase it occupies). Decide where on the precordium it sounds the loudest and where it radiates to and whether or not the intensity varies from the recumbent to the upright position. Practice grading the intensity of the murmur (the same scale is used for children and adults), and ask your preceptor for confirmation.

Innocent murmurs characteristically are **soft** (not louder than grade 3/6, but usually 2/6), **vary in intensity with change in position,** and are associated with **normal S1 and S2 sounds.** Right now, your goal in listening to murmurs in infants, should be to accurately identify the characteristics we have just discussed. After you have accomplished this, you will be able to concentrate on learning to identify the classic innocent and pathologic murmurs. Most innocent murmurs of childhood are easiest to identify in the older toddler on upward. This is partly related to the enhanced cooperation of the older child. You will read more about innocent murmurs in the next chapter.

Finally, identify other adventitious cardiac sounds (e.g., clicks, rubs).

Listen over the anterior and posterior lung fields. Count respiratory rate and observe for increased respiratory effort. Make sure he is aerating well. You should hear air flow during all phases of respiration. Listen for adventitious sounds (crackles, wheezes, or stridor).

The older infant is **very** good at taking deep inspirations but not very good at expirations. How so? By crying. By now, you will be well into your exam. If he has become frightened by the intrusion, don't immediately stop. Take a moment to listen to inspiration, front and back. Then take a few moments to separate yourself from him, allow mom to calm him down, and try a different technique of distraction. When he's calmer, you can try to listen again, paying more attention to the expiratory phases. Crackles are heard mostly during inspiration; these are produced by opening of small previously collapsed airways. Wheezes (from small airway obstruction) are heard more often during expiration, but may be heard during inspiration as well. In order to hear wheezing, the small airways need to be partially open; if they are completely obstructed, breath sounds will be markedly reduced and wheezing may not be heard.[5]

Infants experience many upper respiratory infections (URIs). It takes practice to learn to distinguish auscultated sounds originating in the nose (called "upper airway noises"), from those originating in the lungs. Hold your stethoscope over the nose and compare the sounds that you hear with the lung sounds. This maneuver will help you differentiate these two origins of "noisy breathing" (most of the time the noises are from the upper airway).

Abdomen

The infant's abdomen retains a protruberant shape. The umbilical stump dries, and falls off on average at 1 to 2 weeks after birth. For several more days, the site may ooze small amounts of serous fluid or blood (especially during cleansing). By one month, the site of cord insertion will be covered by new skin. Sometimes, after the cord falls off, a moist, pinkish, greyish stump of granulation tissue (called: an **umbilical granuloma**) is left behind. This may heal by itself or may require cauterization with silver nitrate (an easy, painless, office procedure). If serous fluid continues to drain, consider an abnormal connection between the abdominal surface and the underlying structures (such as a patent urachus). A slight amount of redness surrounding a healing umbilical stump may be present. Increased erythema, foul smell, purulent drainage, or edema all suggest omphalitis, a potentially devastating infection.

Auscultate (making sure stethoscope is warm) for the usual tinkling and gurgling sounds which come in waves approximately 2 to 4 times per minute. With the older infant, make a game of this maneuver (e.g., pretending to hear someone talking inside, smiling, making funny noises). Percussion of the abdomen in infancy is usually peformed only to confirm organomegaly or ascites.

Begin palpation with a very gentle touch. It will be easier for you if the baby is sucking as you do this (e.g., pacifier or bottle). Palpate for organomegaly and masses. A liver edge of 1 to 2 cm. (below the costal margin) is the normal finding; as is a nonpalpable or slightly palpable spleen tip. In the young infant, you will still be able to ballot the kidneys. This becomes more difficult in the older infant, partly because of decreasing cooperation and partly because the abdomen becomes less pliable in the older child. An umbilical hernia may go unnoticed by the parents until the cord falls off. With crying (one way to induce a valsalva maneuver), the lax skin forms an outpouching.

❓ What should you tell the parents about an umbilical hernia? . . . Good, "Don't worry . . . This rarely causes any problems (including obstruction); many disappear within the first two years; if necessary, it can be surgically closed when the baby is older (for cosmetic reasons)."

Inspect and palpate the inguinal areas. A few pea-sized lymph nodes are the rule here too (as in the high cervical areas), especially if there is a diaper rash. Carefully remove the diaper (remember the risk). This is a good time to ask parents of a boy (at the first office visit) if his "stream" is straight and forceful. The answer is usually a resounding yes! Remind yourself to feel the femoral pulse if you haven't done this yet.

Genitalia

Inspect the genitalia and anus carefully.

Female: Inspect the labia majora, then visualize the other structures (clitoris, urethra, vagina, and labia minora) by gently pulling laterally and downwards on the surrounding skin of the perineum. Sometimes, (not at birth) a thin layer of tissue (**labial adhesion**) stretches across the labia minora virtually occluding the vaginal orifice (but allowing a stream of urine to exit the urethra). These labial adhesions may separate or dissipate over time simply from the small degree of trauma associated with diaper changes. Some of the time, adhesions remain until the influence of adolescent estrogen hormone causes them to shrink and break. The physician will occasionally choose to hasten this process by applying local estrogen cream.

❓ If you encounter a vaginal discharge (of blood or mucous) in a 2-week-old, what is the likely cause? Correct . . . It's from the withdrawal of maternal hormones and will resolve during the first month of life. Wait! What else may happen from this phenomenon? Breast engorgement and secretion of "witches milk."

Male: Examine the penis and identify the meatus. Retract the foreskin only as far as it will easily go. The foreskin of a noncircumcised male will not retract too far in infancy. It should become increasingly easier to do this as the child grows. A circumcised male will have an easily visible meatus and glans. During the first few weeks after circumcision, the site of the surgery will remain reddened, and then as healing progresses, there may be some whitish granulation tissue evident. If erythema and tenderness of the glans is prominent, suspect an infection (balanitis).

Palpate the testicles.

❓ What do you do if you cannot feel a testicle in the scrotum? . . . Feel for it along the inguinal canal. If you find it, attempt to "milk" it down into the scrotum. If you don't

find it, palpate the lower abdomen on that side, for a mass.

If you can't feel the testicle easily, put the baby in either a sitting position or a prone position up on all fours. The increased pressure on the lower abdominal contents may make the testicles more palpable or visible.

If there is a bulge in the scrotum, try to discover if there is a hernia or hydrocele. **Transillumination may help!** Many hydroceles resorb during the first 4 to 6 months. After that, if there hasn't been much progress, there isn't likely to be much. That child is likely to have an indirect inguinal hernia and should be referred for surgical repair.

As stated previously, most inguinal hernias in childhood occur in boys, and most of these are of the indirect type. If your history reveals that the parent has seen a bulge in the inguinal area or in the scrotum, but you cannot find it on physical exam, exploring the external ring with your finger (looking for enlargement as you would in an adult) is unlikely to be helpful. The ring is too small to permit your finger to enter it. Feel the spermatic cord for a thickening. Also, rub your finger over the lower part of the inguinal area; if there is a hernia present, it may feel as if you are rubbing two pieces of silk together. This is known as the "silk-glove" sign.

Diaper rashes: The moist, warm and covered groin and buttocks offer the perfect environment for irritant rashes. Add urine and stool, and it's difficult to understand how this area avoids rashes at all! The most common diaper rash is the "generic" one (also called "ammoniacal") (Figure 3.5) from the "contact" of irritating substances. This looks red and dry (almost parchment-like), and usually spares the groin creases.

Once a diaper rash has been present for more than a few days, it often becomes secondarily "infected" by the candida organism. When this happens, the rash becomes "beefy" red, and "satellite" papules develop just beyond the margins.

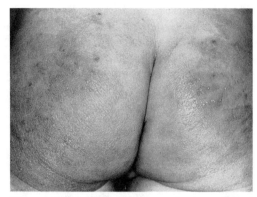

Figure 3.5. Contact diaper rash. Reproduced with permission. Hurwitz S. Clinical pediatric dermatology. Philadelphia: W.B. Saunders, 1981:27. Photo courtesy of Sidney Hurwitz, M.D.

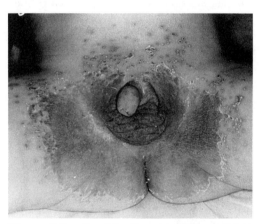

Figure 3.6. Candida diaper rash. Reproduced with permission. Hurwitz, S. Clinical pediatric dermatology. Philadelphia: W.B. Saunders, 1981: 29. Photo courtesy of Sidney Hurwitz, M.D.

❓ What other common lesion does candida produce in the infant? . . . Thrush! If you find thrush, look for candida in the diaper area, too. (The satellite lesions give it away.) A primary candida infection associated with thrush might also be manifested as perianal erythema with satellite lesions.

Diaper rashes may primarily involve the inguinal folds. Earlier, we spoke of intertrigo (nonspecific skin fold irritation). The groin folds may be involved, too. This may also become secondarily infected with candida. The other common skin "ailment" we spoke of was seborrhea. This is difficult to distinguish from intertrigo. A helpful hint is to search for the presence of seborrhea elsewhere. Although there are several other types of diaper rashes, the ones we've mentioned are the most common.

Back

The best time to inspect and palpate the back is when the diaper is off. If you haven't already, look at the posterior neck for webbing or other abnormalities. Run your eyes down the length of the spine, checking for straightness and observe symmetry of scapulae and iliac crests; don't forget to look for posterior thigh fold symmetry, too. The best place to do this is with the infant prone on the examination table. You could also do this while the baby is in mom's lap. However, because the lap isn't a flat surface, an asymmetry may be created simply because the baby isn't lying flat. An apparent asymmetry will have to be re-examined on the table.

Thus far, we've reviewed the exam in a head to toe order, leaving out the intrusive procedures (ears, pharynx, and hips). We're ready to examine the lower extremities (including hips) and preform the neuro-developmental exam (then you will finish with the ears and pharynx). If the baby has remained happy, continue with the exam in the order as written. If the baby is unhappy, attempt to cajole him, skip to the neuro-development section and finish up with the lower extremities (and hips), ears, and pharynx.

Lower Extremities

Parents ask many questions about legs and feet during their child's first few years. These arise especially when the infant begins to stand. More questions surface when the child walks alone, and again when he begins to run. Parents usually focus on the feet: why does his foot (feet) turn in (or out)? You've already begun to prepare to answer these questions by performing a careful orthopedic exam on the newborn. You will now continue your preparation by performing a careful exam on the infant. In the next chapter, you will learn additional maneuvers on the abulating child. Why is it so important to "break down" the lower extremity exam into individual parts? There are several reasons: First, intoeing (or outtoeing) may result from forces at the hip, knee, shaft of the tibia, or foot. Unless you examine these components individually, you will be unable to determine where the "problem" originates, and therefore be unable to answer the question. Second, the "problem" may be physiologic (and self-resolving) rather than pathologic.

With the infant supine, inspect the lower extremities in the same manner as we discussed in the previous chapter. Proceed downwards looking at symmetry of the hip joint, thigh creases, knee alignment, tibiae (which may bow out laterally at the midsection relative to the vertical axis formed by the knee and the foot), ankle alignment, and feet. Move all joints through a range of motion and estimate tone and strength. The flexion contractures of the hips and knees of the newborn disappear within several weeks. Examine the feet with special attention to ruling out metatarsus adductus. It isn't redundant to count toes and inspect for webbing (syndactly), overlapping, or other deformities. Some minor abnormalities (which may not have been discussed thoroughly during the newborn period) may become clinically or cosmetically important as the child prepares to ambulate. At the very least, even if a minor abnormality (e.g., overlapping toe) will not interfere with the initiation of ambulation, it should be reviewed with parents. Counselling by the pediatrician will include discussion of the possibility of future corrective procedures or special footwear requirements.

Examine the hips. On the younger infant (few weeks) perform the Ortolani and Barlow maneuvers. You will continue to examine the hips during the first year, but movement of a dislocated or dislocatable hip, in or out of the acetabulum becomes increasingly difficult after the first month or two of life. Thereafter, the most important part of the hip exam consists of abducting the hips (while they are held in 90° of flexion). The knees should nearly touch the examining table (Figure 3.7). Differences between the two sides are very significant.

By six months, most infants begin to bear weight; that is, when held upright by the arms or under the axillae, the infant will begin to participate actively in maintaining an upright posture. Between nine and twelve months the infant will pull himself upright while holding on to the crib bars and begin to walk while holding on (cruising). The typical stance of the newly upright child has a very wide base; the feet may point in or out (usually slightly outwards relative to direction of forward progression). Parents at this time often ask if their child will always walk "that way." Reassure parents that most children begin to walk with a wide base because it steadies them more than if their legs were close together. As normal development proceeds, the legs come closer together and the feet point straight ahead. If the feet point in because of metatarsus adductus, then stretching exercises or casting will straighten them.

The feet may also point in because of **internal tibial torsion;** in this condition the tibiae are rotated inwards on their longitudinal axis. An easy way to confirm this is to sit the child on the end of the examining table with the knees pointing straight at you (Figure 3.8). Normally, in this position, the malleoli are situated so that the medial malleolus is slightly anterior to the lateral malleolus (or, a little more of the medial malleolus is visible than the lateral malleolus). When the tibia is internally rotated, the lateral malleolus is positioned so that it is more anterior than usual (and the medial malleolus, more posterior than usual). Internal tibial torsion may be bilateral or unilateral. Mild degrees of this condition may resolve without therapy. More significant degrees, a rare occurrence, (such that the deformity looks very obvious or interferes with walking), may be corrected with orthoses: an abduction bar with shoes affixed to it, worn at night and/or daytime twister cables with attached shoes. Other common problems associated with directions of gait will be reviewed in the toddler chapter.

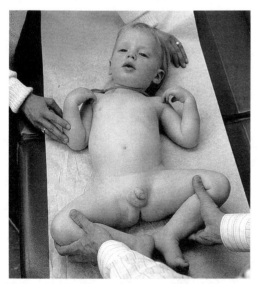

Figure 3.7. Hip abduction exam during infancy; hips should abduct equally, and knees should touch or almost touch the table.

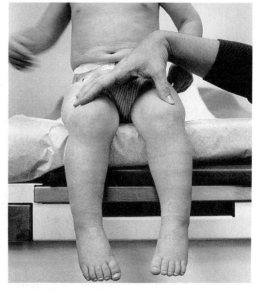

Figure 3.8. Position to inspect for internal tibial torsion.

Neurologic and Development

You've already performed parts of these exams. Now you should mentally review the various components and fill in what you've left out:

General appearance and mental status. The observations we discussed earlier and those you've been making all along apply here (state, transitions of state, alertness, mood, eye contact, consolability). Other parts of the general physical exam that you've already performed are also part of the neurologic exam: growth parameters, examination of the head, spine, skin (for neurocutaneous changes such as cafe au lait spots and depigmented spots), and anomalies or asymmetries.

Review developmental milestones with parents (the history flow sheets will supply you with the age-appropriate ones); confirm these during the physical exam (if possible). Acquisitions of milestones are a gradual process; each child sets his own unique pace; "fits and starts" aren't unusual. Unless there is a consistent "lag" or a blaring omission (or a loss of a previously acquired milestone), lack of attainment of one particular milestone in the context of an otherwise normal exam is probably not significant. If there are multiple problems identified, then further evaluation may be called for. Fatigue, hunger, and fear will affect the results of these maneuvers.

Cranial nerves. Assess as completely as possible. The maneuvers we discussed in the newborn chapter apply in the infant as well.

Motor. Assess bulk, tone and strength. If your patient, by history, hasn't progressed in motor development pay particular attention to tone (floppy or stiff) and strength. Assess tone as the resistance you encounter to passive movement (when the baby is relaxed). Assess strength as the degree of active resistance against you. In addition, information about strength (or weakness) will be supplied as you observe the infant's ability to support his own weight against

gravity (e.g., supporting himself on his elbows, sitting up, and bearing weight). It is more difficult to assess individual muscles in small children, than in adults. Watching infants perform some of their motor "accomplishments" supplies information about muscle **groups** (e.g., head control, rolling over, sitting, bearing weight, and creeping, furnish information about gross motor function; reaching, transferring, banging toys together, furnish information about upper extremity muscles and fine motor function).

A two-week-old will still have substantial head lag when pulled by his arms from the supine to sitting position. A two-month-old will flex his neck a little when he's pulled up and when sitting, his head will bob. In ventral suspension (holding him up in the air, around his waist in the prone position), he will attempt to straighten out his head and legs into the horizontal position. A four-month-old will not have very much head lag when pulled to sit, and his head will not bob; he will partially support his weight when held erect. A six-month-old will have no head lag when pulled to sit; in the sitting position he will lean forward and support himself with his hands on the table (tripoding). A nine-month-old can sit erect for prolonged periods (ten to fifteen minutes).

Coordination. Observation of the infant old enough to reach for or manipulate a small object gives you information about coordination. Balance is observed when the infant sits or tries to walk (remember that this is age-dependent: a "new" achievement is always performed "unsteadily" at first.

Unwanted movements. Observe for tremors (e.g., while watching manipulation of objects), myoclonus (sudden jerking movements) or other abnormal movements.

Sensory. This remains difficult to assess at this young age. Unlike the newborn, the infant is ticklish. If the baby is visually diverted, you may tickle him and see if he responds. Withdrawal to pin or other sensory investigations are best reserved for infants in whom detailed neurologic investigations are required or in whom a true lack of sensation is suspected.

Reflexes.   Deep tendon reflexes (DTRs) may be assessed in a manner similar to adults. You may want to offer an "extra" hammer to the older infant in order to distract him. The magnitude of response in infants may normally be somewhat brisker than you have been used to seeing in adults (e.g., a 3 out of a possible 4 response). Sometimes, you will have difficulty eliciting a DTR in an infant (this is usually an issue of technique, not because the reflex isn't there). You may be more successful tapping gently with your finger, instead of using a hammer. The plantar response is variable at birth and may continue to be variable during the first year of life.

Primitive reflexes.   These supply information about the general state of the neuraxis. Delayed appearance of primitive reflexes or delayed disappearance of primitive reflexes may reflect a problem with neuromaturation. Remember, however, that abnormalities in appearance or disappearance of primitive reflexes are "gross" signs; they aren't specific. Detailed neurologic examination is required to point to more specific areas of dysfunction. Remember, too, that there is a normal spectrum or range in timing. Finally, remember to compare the symmetry of response, as asymmetry may represent paralysis, fracture, etc. of one side.

❓ **What are some of the primitive reflexes in the newborn? . . . Yes: moro, reflex grasp, placing and stepping, root and suck.**

Placing and stepping are present at birth and disappear by approximately 1 to 2 months.

The **moro and reflex grasp** are present at birth; the reflex grasp disappears by approximately age 3 months, and the moro disappears by 6 months (often by 4).

The **tonic neck reflex** (Figure 3.9) is

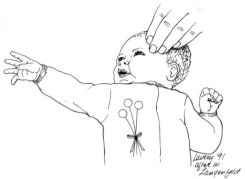

Figure 3.9.   Tonic neck reflex. Adapted with permission. Willms JL, Lewis J. Introduction to clinical medicine. Baltimore: Williams & Wilkins, 1991:146.

variably present at birth, may not appear until sometime during the first month and disappears by approximately age 4 months. This is also called the **fencing posture.** To elicit this (the baby often takes this posture spontaneously): place the baby on his back, and keeping the shoulders level, rotate the head to one side. The extremities on the side the head is facing towards will extend; the opposite extremities will flex. There should not be a striking asymmetry between the tonic neck reflex on one side or the other.

The **parachute reflex** emerges at approximately eight to nine months. To elicit this, hold the infant in ventral suspension and abruptly tilt the baby's head down towards the floor. He will extend both of his arms in a protective manner (Figure 3.10). This reflex never disappears.

Ears and Posterior Pharynx

Examining the ears and the posterior pharynx are the most intrusive parts of infant exam. Adequate visualization (and accurate diagnosis) of the tympanic membranes is also one of the most difficult skills to acquire in pediatric physical diagnosis. "But otitis is so common in kids, I've got to see the eardrums!," reply most of my students after their initial frustrating encounters! It is true that a good pediatrician has to be an "expert" at "ears," but it is also true that it takes a lot of practice to get to that point. So,

Figure 3.10.   Parachute reflex.

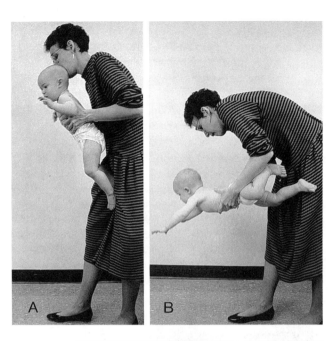

take your time, approach these maneuvers slowly, and don't quit after your first exam. You'll "get it" if you keep trying on each patient.

First, some guidelines:

1. **Proper immobilization is the key to success.** The very young infant who is not yet sitting is probably best examined in the supine position on the examing table. The older infant can either sit in the parent's lap or lie on the table.

These are the methods that work best for me. (If you are left-handed, you can try it this way, or reverse the hand directions if it feels more comfortable): the infant on the examining table should have his arms at his sides. The parent should stand at the baby's feet and lean over him to immobilize the infant's knees (this is key!) with her body and hold the baby's arms down on the table. This frees you to deal only with the baby's head. You can turn the head to either side and restrain it with your left forearm. The left hand is then free to pull back the pinna and the right hand; holding the otoscope can advance it gently into the ear canal. (Figure 3.11)

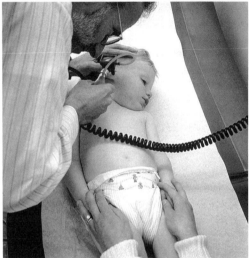

Figure 3.11.   Ear exam using the examination table.

If the child is in the parent's lap, have him sit facing you (you should also be seated), with his legs restrained between the parent's knees. Have the parent wrap one of her arms around and across the infant's arms and chest tightly. With her free hand, she should turn the infant's head to one side and gently restrain it against her chest. This will enable you to use your left hand to pull on the pinna

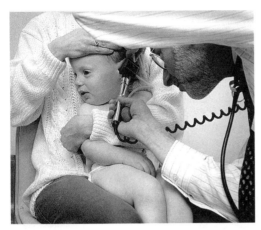

Figure 3.12. Ear exam using the parent's lap.

and your right hand to introduce the otoscope (Figure 3.12).

2. **Use the largest size speculum that will fit in the canal;** in infants the most convenient size is long and narrow (sizes 2.5 or 3).
3. **The infant canal is directed upwards,** so in order to visualize the tympanic membrane at the end of it, the **pinna** should be gently **pulled posteriorly and downwards** as the speculum is advanced.
4. **The shaft of the otoscope should rest in your palm.** (Your hand should always rest against the child's head, separating the head from the shaft of the otoscope). Thus, if the infant moves suddenly, he will push against your hand, which in turn, controls the depth of penetration of the speculum. This reduces the potential for injury with a struggling infant.
5. The otoscope should be equipped with a connecting tube and a rubber bulb at the end of it (**a pneumatic otoscope**). With the otoscope shaft resting in your palm, place the bulb against the outer side of the shaft and hold it in place under your thumb (Figure 3.13).
6. With the older infant and toddler, make whispered noises as you insert and advance the otoscope into the canal. Sometimes this is enough of a distractor that the infant will forget to cry.
7. Gently advance the otoscope head into the canal as you look through the head. The canal is normally pink or flesh colored. Drainage from a ruptured tympanic membrane (purulent-appearing) or cerumen ("wax": orange, yellow, or brown) may obscure the tympanic membrane. You may need to ask for assistance from a more experienced person in clearing the cerumen. If it is soft and easily visible and you feel confident of the ability of the parent to cooperate in restraining the child, you may wish to attempt to clear the cerumen. Use the special currette devised for this purpose (it has a metal loop at the end of it). Under excellent visualization only, "scoop" out the cerumen; taking care to avoid the friable tissue of the canal; and avoid going deeper than you can see (and risking injury to the tympanic membrane).
8. The normal tympanic membrane is light grey in color, semi-transparent and slanted away from the examiner. The normal landmarks are shown below. (Figure 3.14) You may need to change

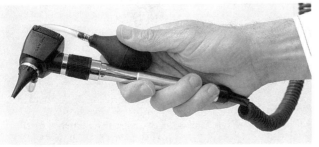

Figure 3.13. The pneumatic otoscope.

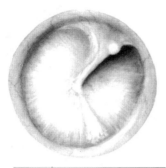

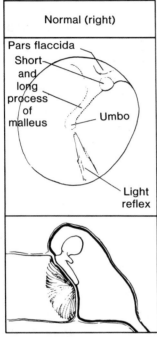

Figure 3.14. Normal tympanic membrane. Reproduced with permission. Fleisher GR, Ludwig S, eds. Textbook of pediatric emergency medicine. 2nd ed. Baltimore: Williams & Wilkins, 1988:428.

canal in young infants sometimes moves with insufflation). Like visualizing the TM, learning what the "normal" amount of movement is, takes lots of practice. It also takes a good "seal" with the speculum and the canal. **Changing to a larger size speculum may be necessary in order to obtain a good seal.**

If you are extremely gentle, sometimes the baby will not cry. If he does (and it doesn't mean you've failed), the tympanic membranes will redden. If the landmarks all

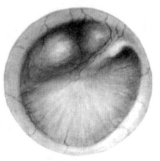

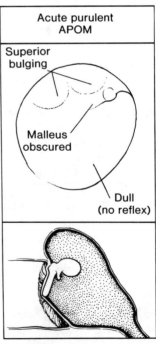

Figure 3.15. Acute purulent otitis media. Reproduced with permission. Fleisher GR, Ludwig S, eds. Textbook of pediatric emergency medicine. 2nd ed. Baltimore: Williams & Wilkins, 1988:428.

the angle of your otoscope in order to visualize the entire tympanic membrane (TM).

9. **Once you have visualized the TM, push in gently on the bulb and then release it.** The TM should move in as you push against the bulb and then return outwards to its initial position as you release it. If you see movement, make sure it's the drum that's moving, not the canal (the external surface of the

appear normal, and the drums move in and out with insufflation, and there is equal redness on both sides, then the redness is probably related to vascular engorgement (from crying) and not to infection.

Infection of the middle ear, (otitis media) causes the TM to appear increasingly opaque and reddened. The normal landmarks behind the TM become progressively more obscured by purulent fluid (either yellow or white). The drum itself may look very red, or have patches of red. As fluid accumulates behind the drum, it begins to bulge out towards you (Figure 3.15). The more fluid that accumulates, the less the drum will move in response to insufflation. If this is a routine child health maintenance visit, and the baby has been asymptomatic (not febrile, fussy, or with other signs of illness), it is still possible for him to have acute otitis media. The ability of some infants to tolerate an acute otitis without symptoms always amazes me. This is one of the reasons (there are others we'll discuss in other chapters) it is so important for you to learn to adequately visualize the TM. Further observations of the ear canal and tympanic membrane will be discussed in later chapters.

Finally, you need to "catch" a glimpse of the posterior pharynx. If the infant is crying, shine your otoscope light into the mouth (or grab a flashlight and do the same).

If you don't have that opportunity and the infant is supine on the table, change places with the parent. Have her stand at the baby's head. Ask her to bring her baby's arms up over his head, so that they rest against his ears; restrain the arms against the head. You stand at the baby's feet and lean over him to immobilize his lower body (this way both your hands are free). Hold your light source in one hand and the tongue depressor in the other hand. Attempt to gently tease open the mouth with the tongue depressor; work the stick gently back into the mouth while pressing down on the tongue (a side-to-side rotation of your wrist usually works best). Depress the tongue; eventually you will trigger a gag reflex; Take a good, quick look; for well children, that's all the time you need. (Figure 3.16)

If the infant is in mom's lap, have her restrain his arms by wrapping one of her arms across his chest. Have her, using her other hand, press against his forehead to restrain the head against her chest. (Figure 3.17)

Inspect gums, tongue, buccal mucosa, palate, uvula, tonsils, and posterior pharynx. Don't assume a thorough job of inspecting for congenital anomalies was done in the newborn period. Do it again.

Look for redness, bumps, lumps, and ulcers. You may see mucus drainage in the posterior pharynx (postnasal drip seen in upper respiratory infections, otitis media,

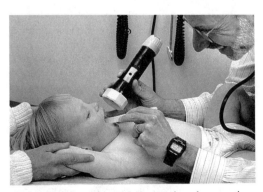

Figure 3.16. Pharynx exam using the examination table.

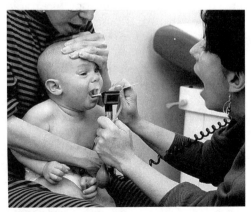

Figure 3.17. Pharynx exam using the parent's lap.

and sinusitis). The tonsils are small in infancy but may redden or have a white or yellow exudate in the presence of an upper respiratory infection. The uvula may also become erythematous and/or swollen when there is a respiratory infection.

❓ If the uvula is bifid, what is the child at risk for? (This is to remind you to continue to look for and think about congenital anomalies, even "asymptomatic" ones, during *every* exam.) The child is at risk for speech and hearing difficulties. If you find a bifid uvula, don't forget to palpate for a submucous cleft of the soft palate; the bifid uvula may be a marker for that hidden problem.

If your patient has stridor or respiratory distress, do not attempt to force his mouth open; ask for help in evaluating him. Infectious causes of stridor include viral croup and bacterial epiglotittis. Children with epiglotittis are especially vulnerable to sudden airway obstruction; forced pharyngeal examination may initiate this.

There are several variations of normal appearance of the tongue which concern parents. Geographic tongue, in which the surface has the appearance of a relief map, may be normal or signal underlying allergic disease. Scrotal tongue, in which there are deep furrows, has no significance. Tremors of the tongue are seen in some neurologic and neuromuscular diseases.

Once your inspection of the posterior aspect of the mouth is finished, allow the mom to comfort her infant immediately. Move away from the patient. Once he's calmed down, smile at him from a distance. Your "invasive" physical exam is over. If you need to perform any painful tests (e.g., blood drawing or immunizations), you'll run the unavoidable risk of antagonizing him again. If you are lucky enough to be done at this point, chances are if you can reward the older infant with a little toy or even a smile, you'll manage to make friends again.

CLINICAL ASSESSMENT OF THE ILL INFANT

THE PROBLEM: "JUANITA'S BEEN CRYING ALL NIGHT"

It's nine A.M. on a bright spring morning. You're having your second cup of coffee with your outpatient "team" while discussing some issues that came up on "work rounds" in the newborn nursery. Ellen, the nurse in the outpatient department appears in the conference room, bearing a sheet of progress note paper, stamped with the name of a patient. The look on her face says: "This shouldn't wait too long." Scheduled health care maintenance and routine problem visits don't ordinarily begin until 9:30; this signals a more pressing problem.

"It's Juanita Rodriguez," Ellen says. "She's a patient of ours, who's seven months old. She was up all night crying. She's had a fever all night, but now her temperature is 100°F. Her mom gave her acetaminophen an hour ago. Her old chart is on its way, but she's been pretty healthy up until now."

You are still pretty new at this, but you're eager. You get up, grab your stethoscope and take the paper from Ellen. You remember to take along the infancy history flow sheet. She points towards the examining room and says, "Just yell if you need a hand." (You think to yourself, "I need more than a hand!") Before you enter the room, you glance at the "6 month" flow columns and wonder how "heavily" into stranger and separation anxiety little Juanita is (hoping she's a little slow!).

As you enter cautiously, you see Juanita lying in her mother's arms sleeping. She's wearing a diaper and undershirt. You introduce yourself quietly and take a history:

Juanita was well until two days ago when she developed a runny nose and a slight cough. The mucus from her nose was clear initially. Yesterday, she began to get fussier and refuse her cereal. She nursed more frequently than usual (every few hours), but only sucked for a few minutes at a time. Last night, she developed a fever of 103° and spent most of the night needing to be comforted in her mother's arms. She slept in short intervals. She vomited once. She had two stools yesterday which were a little looser than normal. She wet six diapers (normal for her).

Her past medical history is unremarkable. She has been a healthy child up until now; her growth and development are normal. She is normally a happy, smiley baby. She has begun to cry when she sees strangers come close ("Oh, great!" you say to yourself.) There are several children in her day care group that have colds.

You quietly move over to mom's chair and begin to warm up the diaphragm of your stethoscope. You plan to try to listen to her chest without waking her.

❓ What have you forgotten? Right! Wash your hands.

Unfortunately, the sound of the running water wakes Juanita and she starts to cry. She takes one look at you and the volume of her cry increases dramatically. Large pools of tears run down her face. You retreat back to your chair and make sympathetic noises. Mrs. Rodriguez comforts Juanita and asks if you'd mind if she nursed her for a minute. Why should you mind? Anything to calm her down! Juanita settles down after a brief interval and begins to suck eagerly.

While she sucks, you notice that her skin is nice and pink, without mottling or cyanosis. After a few minutes of sucking, she stops and looks around. Her mom continues to make eye contact with her and comfort her. She sits her up in her lap and pulls out her very favorite stuffed doggy and puts it into Juanita's hands. Juanita immediately puts it into her mouth and sucks on it.

You try approaching again, by wheeling your chair over slowly. This time, Juanita looks at you suspiciously, but continues to suck on her animal. You warm your stethoscope again. Mrs. Rodriguez lifts up Juanita's shirt so you can get to her chest. This time, you are more successful. You feel her precordium and then listen. By stopping each time Juanita looks a little worried and making some funny noises with your mouth and smiling all the while you are able to examine her heart and her lungs. You hear some upper airway noises, but otherwise her lung and heart exams are normal.

You perform the rest of the exam in mom's lap and find:

Her pulse is 100; Her respiratory rate is 25. Skin color and turgor are normal. Her anterior fontanelle is flat but not sunken. Her eyes are not injected or sunken. There is a small amount of crusting at the left inner canthus, and the skin below that is slightly reddened. Her mom tells you it always looks like that.

❓ What's the most likely cause of the recurrent crusting at the medial canthus?

Yes! Congenital nasolacrimal duct obstruction.

The rest of her eye exam is normal. Her nose is dripping yellow mucus. The mucosa is reddened. There is some erythema just below her nares. You decide to skip the ears and mouth for now.

Her neck is supple. (Remember, at this age, nuchal rigidity may be absent even in the presence of meningeal irritation.) There are a few, slightly enlarged lymph nodes in the anterior cervical areas on both sides. These are soft, nontender, freely mobile nodes.

Her abdomen is soft, nontender, without organomegaly or masses. You pick up a small fold of abdominal skin and as you release it, it springs back easily. Her skin turgor is normal. If she was severely dehydrated, her skin would not spring back immediately; it would remain "tented" up. In some children with dehydration (hypernatremic dehydration) the skin has a "doughy" feel to it. You hear occasional tinkling bowel sounds. Her inguinal areas and genitalia appear and feel normal, except for a few shoddy inguinal nodes bilaterally, too. There is a diffuse, dry, red diaper rash sparing the skin folds.

Even though Juanita hasn't smiled at you, she's allowed you to do most of your exam so far. When you show Mrs. Rodriguez how to restrain her for the ear exam (with Juanita in her lap), she starts to cry. ("Oh, great! Now her eardrums will be red!") You decide to get this over with, and examine her ears and her throat.

Wow! Both tympanic membranes are bright red. There is a yellow discoloration behind both drums; you cannot see any landmarks, and the drums move only slightly upon insufflation. By now, Juanita is crying vigorously, so you peer into her throat. Her posterior pharynx is slightly reddened and there is some yellow mucus coating it.

You've just made your first diagnosis of bilateral acute otitis media! You tell mom what you've found. Mrs. Rodriguez sighs, and begins to calm Juanita down. Juanita wants to nurse again. When she stops nursing, she gives her mom a brief smile. You tell Mrs. Rodriguez you'll be back shortly. You go back to the conference room to report your findings to your resident.

Your resident, Cathy, listens to your presentation. She smiles and says: "See, I told you it wasn't so hard. But you left out a few impressions. Tell me about her state of hydration."

You think to yourself, "What do I know about

Table 3.2
Acute Illness Observation Scales

Observation Item	1 Normal	3 Moderate Impairment	5 Severe Impairment
Quality of cry	Strong with normal tone OR Content and not crying	Whimpering OR Sobbing	Weak OR Moaning OR High pitched
Reaction to parent stimulation	Cries briefly then stops OR Content and not crying	Cries off and on	Continual cry OR Hardly responds
State variation	If awake → stays awake OR If asleep and stimulated → wakes up quickly	Eyes close briefly → awake OR Awakes with prolonged stimulation	Falls to sleep OR Will not rouse
Color	Pink	Pale extremities OR Acrocyanosis	Pale OR Cyanotic OR Mottled OR Ashen
Hydration	Skin normal, eyes normal AND Mucous membranes moist	Skin, eyes-normal AND Mouth slightly dry	Skin doughy OR Tented AND Dry mucous membranes AND/OR Sunken eyes
Response (talk, smile) to social overtures	Smiles OR Alerts (≤2 mo)	Brief smile OR Alerts briefly (≤2 mo)	No smile Face anxious, dull, expressionless OR No alerting (≤2 mo)

Used with permission from McCarthy PL, Sharpe MR, Spiesel SZ, et al. Observation scales to identify serious illness in febrile children. *Pediatrics* 1982;70:802–9.

that?" Well, in fact, you know quite a bit: Skin turgor was normal, and her eyes and anterior fontanelle weren't sunken. (But those may not be helpful signs until significant dehydration has occurred. Rapid heart rate and low blood pressure might also be expected.) What else? Lips, tongue, and mucous membranes were moist. She cried tears freely. Her mom said that she had wet 6 diapers the day before (same as usual). These are more helpful parameters in judging milder (3–5%) degrees of dehydration. Juanita isn't dehydrated.

Next, Cathy asks you how ill Juanita appears. You're not sure how to answer her, besides repeating your findings on physical exam. Cathy explains: "When evaluating an infant or toddler with a febrile illness, it's important to try and assess "toxicity." For years, pediatricians, using their clinical "gestalt," have recognized that a febrile child who appears "very ill" or "toxic" is more likely to have a serious illness than those who do not have this appearance. This "gestalt" has now been quantified into observational

scales. One of the most widely accepted is called the Acute Illness Observation Scales (AIOS).[6] We now know that "observational assessment using the AIOS and done prior to the history and physical, with the child seated comfortably on the parent's lap, provides additional sensitivity to the traditional clinical evaluation."[7] The data from the studies using the AIOS gives credence to what pediatricians have long appreciated intuitively.[8] These scales are used in children less than 24 months (and especially between 6 and 24 months). Very young infants (especially 3 months and under) are much more difficult to assess clinically for toxicity (signs of toxicity may not be as reliable). In this age group, pediatricians are more likely to add laboratory investigations to aid them in their decision-making process.

The AIOS is composed of six items shown above on the left hand column. Each item has a 3 point scale: 1 = normal, 3 = moderate impairment, 5 = severe impairment. The best possible score on the AIOS is 6 (item) x 1 (normal) = 6.

The worst possible score is 30. On the basis of studies performed using the AIOS, a score greater than 10 indicates ill appearance.[6]

Cathy says, "Now, review your observations of this patient." You respond, "her cry was strong; she stopped crying when comforted by her mom; her color was pink; she was normally hydrated; she smiled at her mom only briefly. That last observation was the only abnormal one. So, she gets a 3 for that, and a 1 for everything else. That makes her total score: an 8—not high enough to qualify as "ill appearance."

You accompany Cathy back into the room to confirm your findings and write out a prescription for antibiotics. Cathy also gives Mrs. Rodriguez some guidelines to follow to assist her in judging Juanita's progress. You note that these guidelines include some of the observational assessments that you just spoke about.

Don't memorize the numbers involved in the AIOS. At this point in your training, the observation items and range of findings should serve as a teaching tool in learning to assess "toxicity." This also should remind you of what has been emphasized throughout this text: **In clinical encounters with well or sick children observation is your most powerful clinical ally.**

References

1. Solomon R. Pediatric experiences in year II clinical sciences. E. Lansing, Michigan: Department of Pediatrics and Human Development, College of Human Medicine, Michigan State University, 1986.
2. Moss JR. Helping young children cope with the physical examination. Pediatr Nurs 1981;March/April:19.
3. Athreya BH, Silverman BK. Pediatric Physical Diagnosis. Norwalk, Connecticut: Appleton-Century-Crofts, 1985:92.
4. Von Noorden GK. Binocular Vision and Ocular Motility. St. Louis: C.V. Mosby Co., 1980.
5. Cloutier M. Pulmonary diseases. In: Dworkin PH, ed. The national medical series for independent study: Pediatrics. New York: John Wiley & Sons, Inc., 1987.
6. McCarthy PL, Sharpe MR, Spiesel SZ, et al. Observation scales to identify serious illness in febrile children. Pediatrics 1982;70:802–809.
7. McCarthy PL, Lembo RM, Fink HD, Baron MA, Cicchetti DV. Observation, history and physical examination in diagnosis of serious illness in febrile children ≤24 months. J Pediatr 1987;110:29.
8. McCarthy PL, Lembo RM, Fink HD, Baron MA, Cicchetti DV. Observation, history and physical examination in diagnosis of serious illness in febrile children ≤24 months. J Pediatr 1987;110:30.

CHAPTER **4**

Toddler

THE TODDLER HISTORY
Student Task

1. Obtain a toddler history.

The young toddler will be your toughest customer.[1] His intense parental attachment and fear of strangers are challenges for the best of us. Now I've put you off. Wait! I said tough, not impossible.

By now you should remember the routine:

Preparation
Observation
Modification

Review the old chart. Find out the purpose of the visit. Plot measurements. Review the flow sheet columns for age-appropriate questions and observations to make. By reviewing the developmental agendas and milestones, you also arm yourself with plans for deterring fears.

By the way, there is one encouraging note. The older toddler (three and four) will reward you for your efforts by wanting to be your friend!

As you knock and cautiously open the door, you're just in time to observe Mrs. Dodd giving 18-month-old David a resounding smack on his hand. She says: "Don't touch that outlet again!" David starts to scream and hit wildly at his mother. You feel like saying: "Maybe I should come back later." But you know you can't, so you continue inside and look for the farthest chair. Mrs. Dodd scoops David up into her arms, grabs a ragged blanket off the table and says: "Now David, that's dangerous! Calm down, you'll be o.k." David pops his

thumb into his mouth and clutches the blanket as his sobs diminish. He notices you and looks away. Not exactly an auspicious beginning.

You look away from David as you introduce yourself. You identify Mrs. Dodd and David, and review the purpose of the visit. David is here for a health maintenance visit.

In this short interaction you've already gotten quite a bit of information.

❓ **What *observations* have you made about this toddler/mother dyad? You've observed David's negativism (*autonomy/independence*) and his lack of impulse control. You've deduced that he is inquisitive (*temperament and cognitive development*). You know something about his mother's style of discipline (*temperament*). He sucks his thumb (*habits*) and has a security blanket ("lovey"). If you were quick, you observed his gait (*motor development*). You are confident that he is afraid of strangers and attached to his mom (*attachment*). This is all probably beginning to seem obvious to you. If so, then you're learning to use *observation* to obtain important information.**

As you begin to find out more about David, you set out: blocks, a doll, 2 toy cars, your tongue stick, and stethoscope on the table in front of David and his mother. Your preparations will pay off. Continue to ignore him, as he isn't yet ready for more direct interaction with you. You are friendly and soft spoken with Mrs. Dodd. You smile a lot. As you gather more history you bring your chair slightly closer to the two of them, continuing to avoid direct eye contact with David.

Toddler History Flow Sheets

Below are the history flow sheets for toddlers, with explanatory notes. Familiarize yourself with their contents, although memorization isn't necessary.

Young Toddler Explanatory Notes: (Fifteen Months Through Two Years)

During the second year, conflicts regarding autonomy and independence pervade many aspects of daily life. As the toddler struggles to exert control, the potential for battles is enormous. When limit-setting by caretakers is too restrictive, the child rebels at meal times, bed time, and most hours in between. When limit-setting is absent and the toddler gains the "upper hand," chaos reigns. Neither situation is optimal. A child does best when his parents understand his temperamental style and developmental abilities. A "good fit" between parents and child is achieved with a balance between flexibility and limit setting. **As you obtain the toddler history,** don't just ask specific questions about the various items in the flow sheets. Ask parents about expecta-

Table 4.1
History Flow Sheets: Toddler

	History			Interval Updates	
Early Toddler	General Care	Growth and Development	Developmental Milestones	General Health (ROS and PMH)	Family and Psycho-Social
Fifteen Months	Feeding cup, spoon weaning ↓ intake Sleep pattern difficulties Elimination training deferred Safety toddler car seat aspiration poisons Dental tooth care bottle in bed avoided Shoes purposes	Affective Temperament parental assessment discipline style Attachment Autonomy/ Independence visibility of struggle tantrums/ "me want" negativism Physical Motor concerns with legs/ feet Growth rate slowing	Walks alone Pincer grasp- neat Bangs 2 blocks Scribbles spontaneously MaMa/DaDa specific Indicates wants	Health Update Screening t.b. test reaction Immunization reactions contraindi- cations Vision/hearing	Family status employment update day care
Eighteen Months	Feeding negativism refusals Sleep issues Elimination toilet training: readiness Safety auto/street poisons Toys "lovey"/parent reaction symbolic play	Affective Temperament parental assessment Attachment heightened stranger anxiety Autonomy/ Independence negativism Cognitive representation	Descends stairs alone ± throws ball overhand turns pages uses spoon piles 2 blocks identifies body part 3 new words	Health update Immunization reactions contraindications Habits thumbsucking pica Vision/hearing	Family status

Table continued

Table 4.1—*continued*

	History			Interval Updates	
Early Toddler	General Care	Growth and Development	Developmental Milestones	General Health (ROS and PMH)	Family and Psycho-Social
Two Years	Feeding issues Sleep issues Elimination toilet training Safety auto/street poison control Toys/Play parallel/selfish Dental tooth care/ parental participation	Affective Temperament Attachment separation problems Autonomy/ Independence Impulse Control abilities, parental expectations Cognitive "what's this"? Physical rate of change motor degree of activity rough & tumble play	Climbs stairs unaided Kicks ball Piles 4 blocks Holds cup securely Use of pronouns mine, me, you, I	Health Update Vitamins/ Fluoride dosage Screening lead screen result Immunization reactions contraindications Habits masturbation Poison control ipecac phone # Vision/hearing	Family Status
Older Toddler					
Three Years	Feeding issues/diet Sleep pattern, issues Elimination bowel/bladder control Safety street supervision pets carseat/ shoulder belt Play preferences T.V. violence Dental 1st visit	Affective Temperament parental assessment Attachment Autonomy/ Independence separation Impulse control abilities/ parental expectations Peer interaction sharing nursery school Cognitive language mastery questioning	Pedals trike Copies ○ Vertical line imitate Shares playthings Picture book "what is . . . doing"?	Health Update Vitamins/ Fluoride dosage Immunization reactions contraindications Habits Vision parental perception readiness for formal screen Hearing parental perception Speech intelligibility (50–75%) concerns	Family Status Sibling rivalry

Table 4.1—*continued*

	History			Interval Updates	
Older Toddler	General Care	Growth and Development	Developmental Milestones	General Health (ROS and PMH)	Family and Psycho-Social
Four Years	Feeding issues/diet snacks Sleep pattern, issues Elimination bowel/bladder control Safety playground strangers Play television restrictions	Affective Temperament parental assessment Autonomy/ Independence separation Impulse control ↑ control parental expectations ↑ demands Peer interaction Gender identity Cognitive school readiness parental expectations child's feeling phys/child relationship	Body parts points Heel walking Finger opposition Copies ○ Digit span 5-2-1-6 (one error) General knowledge Name, age, address (2 out of 3)	Health Update Immunization reactions contraindications Habits Vision parental perception readiness for formal screen Hearing parental perception readiness for formal screen Speech intelligibility concerns	Family Status

tions for their child and for an assessment of their child's temperamental style. **In other words, obtain information which ultimately will enable you to estimate what the "goodness of fit" is between the various household members.**

GENERAL CARE

Feeding

Does the child use a cup and a spoon?. Is weaning (from breast or bottle) occurring? Are there difficulties with weaning? Is mealtime a time of conflict and food refusal? How is this handled? What does the child eat in the course of a day? Is intake dramatically less than during the first year? How much milk, juice, and water does he drink?

Sleeping

What is the child's typical sleep pattern (day and night)? Does the child have difficulty falling asleep or staying asleep? How are problems approached?

Elimination

Has the child shown signs of toilet training readiness? (e.g., Does he desire to: use a potty, please his parents, imitate adults, obtain autonomy; Does he have the ability to sit on a potty and walk well? This doesn't usually occur until age 18–24 months.)[2] If toilet training has begun, what methods are used, and what are the results?

Safety

Ask a general question regarding safety measures taken both in and out of the house. Does he use a car seat? How is the ambulating child supervised in the street? What measures have been taken to prevent poisonings? Are foods and toys that may be aspirated avoided? (e.g., nuts, hot dogs, popcorn, small toys).

Toys

What types of toys does the toddler play with? Does he enjoy "pretend" play (symbolic play)? Does he have a special object ("lovey") (e.g., blanket or toy) that he uses for comfort? What is the parent's reaction to this? Does the toddler mostly prefer playing by himself or with a parent? Is he unwilling to share? What is the parental reaction to these age-appropriate patterns of play?

Dental

Does the baby take a bottle to bed? If so what liquid is in it? Does the two-year-old use a toothbrush under supervision?

Shoes

Does the child wear shoes? How often? What type does he wear?

GROWTH AND DEVELOPMENT
Affective Development

Temperament: What are parents' assessments of the child's behavioral style? (e.g., easy, difficult, outgoing, inquisitive, etc.) How do the parents feel about this? How is the child disciplined?

Attachment: What is the child's reaction to strangers? How does the child separate from his parents? How are problems handled?

Autonomy/Independence: Does the toddler exhibit negativism, temper tantrums, breath holding spells, "me want," or other visible expressions of the struggle for independence? How are these handled by parents?

Impulse Control: What are the child's abilities to control his impulses? Does this differ from parental expectations? How is "out of control" behavior handled?

Cognitive Development

Does the child "pretend"? Does he seem to understand about things or persons that are not actually present (representation)? Does the two-year-old ask "what's this"?

Physical Development

Motor: Is the child "always on the go?" Are there concerns about his walking? Are parents worried about the appearance of his feet or legs? Does the two-year-old enjoy "rough housing?"

Growth: Has his growth rate noticeably slowed?

DEVELOPMENTAL MILESTONES

Does the fifteen-month-old walk well? Does he pick up small objects using his thumb and forefinger (pincer grasp)? If he is given two blocks will he bang them together? If given a crayon, will he scribble? Does he say "momma" or "dadda" in the appropriate context? Does he indicate that he wants something by some method other than crying?

Does the eighteen-month-old go down the stairs by himself? Can he throw a ball overhand? (he may not yet be able to do this). Does he like to turn the pages of a book? Can he use a spoon? If given two blocks, can he pile one on top of another (if this is demonstrated)? Can he point to a body part when it is named? Does he say three words other than "mama" or "dada?"

Does the two-year-old walk up the stairs by himself? Can he kick a ball? If given blocks, can he make a "tower" of at least four blocks? Does he hold a cup well? Does he use pronouns such as: "mine," "me," "you," or "I?"

GENERAL HEALTH

Obtain an interval update.

Vitamins/Fluoride

Review vitamin and fluoride dosage and use.

Screening

Review results of recent screening (e.g., lead, tuberculin).

Immunizations

If immunizations are scheduled, review patient and household contraindications. This includes reviewing reactions to prior immunizations.

Habits

Does the toddler suck his fingers or thumb or exhibit any other habits or self-soothing behavior? When does he do it? What are the parents' reactions to this? Does he routinely place nonfood items in his mouth (pica)? Does he masturbate? How do parents respond?

Poison Control

Is poison control phone number readily available in household? Is there a bottle of ipecac in the house? Do parents know what to do in the event of an ingestion?

Vision/Hearing

Does the child seem to see and hear well?

FAMILY/PSYCHO-SOCIAL

Obtain an interval update. Any problems? How is everyone doing? Is everyone healthy? Review parent-child and sibling relationships. Review employment situations. Review home situation (e.g., who is living in the household, etc.). What are the daycare arrangements?

Older Toddler Explanatory Notes (Three and Four Years)

GENERAL CARE

Feeding

What does the toddler's diet consist of? Are there concerns related to food or meals? What snacks are offered and in what quantity? .

Sleep

What is the toddler's pattern? How are problems dealt with?

Elimination

What is the toddler's pattern? Has day/night control and bowel/bladder control been achieved yet? Are there issues surrounding training?

Safety

Does the child use a car seat? If over 40 pounds, does the child wear a shoulder harness seat belt? What type of supervision is there for outdoor play? Has instruction about crossing streets and driveways begun? Has there been a discussion about interacting with strangers? Is playground free of avoidable injury-producing equipment and hazards? Has instruction about "safe play" with pets begun?

Play

What type of play does the toddler prefer? How much television time is allowed? Are there restrictions placed on the type of programs watched?

Dental

Has the three-year-old visited the dentist?

GROWTH AND DEVELOPMENT
Affective Development

Temperament: What is the child's behavioral style, and is it usually predictable? How do the parents feel about it?

Attachment: What is the child's reaction to strangers? This remains an important agenda and should be discussed especially for the three-year-old.

Autonomy/Independence: What is the toddler's ability to separate from his parents? If he attends preschool, has the issue of separation been a problem? How is it handled?

Impulse Control: The three-year-old may still exhibit difficulties in controlling his "aggressions." What are the areas of greatest conflict? How are these handled? The four-year-old has more societal demands made on him. Is increasing ability to control his impulses visible? What are the problem areas? How are these handled? Are rules at home consistent with those at preschool or daycare?

Peer Interaction: How does the toddler relate to other children? Does he share his things sometimes? Are there problems? If so, how have these been handled? Does the child go to preschool? How is that going?

Gender Identity: Does the child enjoy imitating or dressing in clothes of the opposite sex? How do the parents react to this age appropriate behavior?

Cognitive Development

During this period of preoperational development, language becomes increasingly sophisticated. Does the three-year-old ask lots of "why do I have to . . ." questions? How do the parents respond to these?

At the four-year visit, both parental and child reactions to approaching school entry should be explored. What are the parent's perceptions of the child's school readiness (especially around the areas of separation and readiness to do schoolwork)?

The physician will want to increase his or her direct communication with the toddler during history taking and later during examination. Questions about "school," "lunch," riding a "bike," and general knowledge may be addressed directly to the patient. This will not only supply information about the patient's life, but will also supply information about the child's cognitive skills and language development. It also sets the tone for future increasing direct patient-physician interaction.

DEVELOPMENTAL MILESTONES

Does the three-year-old ride a tricycle? Can he crudely copy a circle and a vertical line? Does he share playthings sometimes? Does he enjoy looking at a picture book and being asked "What is . . . doing?"

Does the four-year-old correctly point to body parts such as the waist, knee, nose, and heel? Can he walk on his heels a distance of about 6 feet? Can he imitate the examiner's rapid finger opposition of thumb and fore-finger? Can he crudely copy a drawing of two circles atop one-another? Can he repeat a 4 digit span with only one sequential error? Can he correctly answer 2 out of 3 questions relating to: name, age, and address?

GENERAL HEALTH

Obtain an interval update.

Vitamins/Fluoride

Review vitamin and fluoride dosage and use.

Immunizations

If immunizations are scheduled, review patient and household contraindications. This includes reviewing reactions to prior immunizations.

Habits

Does the toddler have any "habits?" When does he engage in these? What are parents' reactions? Does he have pica? How is masturbation handled?

Vision

Does the child seem to see well? Is the child ready to understand and follow directions for an objective vision screening test? Does the child discriminate any colors correctly?

Hearing

Does the child seem to hear well? If the child is four, is he ready to cooperate and follow directions for an objective hearing test?

Speech

Is the three-year-old's speech 50 to 75% intelligible? Is most of the four-year-old's speech intelligible? Does the toddler exhibit speech patterns such as letter substitutions, hesitancies, or stuttering? What is the pattern? When was this first noticeable? How often does the toddler exhibit this pattern? How do the parents react when their child does this? How do the parents feel about it? You will read more about speech patterns in the physical exam.

Obtain an interval update. Any problems? How is everyone doing? Is everyone healthy? Review parent-child relationships. Review sibling relationships and inquire about sibling rivalry. Have there been any recent major changes in the household?

THE PHYSICAL EXAM OF THE TODDLER

Student Task

1. Examine a toddler.

General Approach[1]

During your conversation with Mrs. Dodd, David (remember: 18 months) gradually calms down. He remains in the protective web of his mother and his blanket but has managed to turn his body towards the table in front of them. He can't resist looking at, and gingerly reaching out towards, the many interesting objects you have placed there. You observe him out of the corner of your eye but continue to **avoid direct eye contact.** As you speak, you **gradually draw your chair closer** to him until it is almost next to him. This position, rather than directly across from him, may be less threatening.[3] When eye contact is made briefly, you smile tentatively, but continue speaking to Mrs. Dodd. At first, David looks away. You pick up the toy car and roll it towards him on the table top. David follows the car, looks at you, (you nod encouragingly), and picks up the car. He begins to play with it. You pick up the second car and begin to roll it back and forth. David looks back at you and reaches for the second car. You hand it to him and allow him some time to play as you conclude the initial history with Mrs. Dodd.

See what's happened? You've taken your time. You've **prepared** for predictable fears

(separation and stranger anxiety), **observed** a child's reaction, state, and developmental level, and **modified** your physical approach, gaze, and voice accordingly. This allows him time to get used to you and your surroundings.[4]

You've done well so far. But remember, David is no easy customer. You still haven't touched him! Before this happens, don't forget to wash your hands. When you get up to do this, back your chair away first. **Announce** what you're going to do (toddlers are very concrete). **Avoid sudden (likely to frighten) movements.**[3] Make a big deal of turning on the water (toddlers love water). Invite him to wash his hands too. If you're lucky, he'll be interested and brave. Once you are done, return to your seat and play a moment longer, rather than "bursting" into the exam.

Measurements

If you haven't already, this is a good time to plot length (or standing height) and weight on the growth charts.

❓ **Should you measure the head circumference in this eighteen-month-old healthy child? . . . That's right, after age one, head circumference is measured only in a new patient or if there are special concerns about head growth, general growth or neurologic problems.**

David may now allow you to play with him directly, at first using a car or blocks to intervene between you. You're performing his general neurologic assessment and observing his fine motor skills. Perhaps by now he has even deigned to try out his few words on you. Assessing his development and the parts of the neurologic exam that require observation are nonthreatening ways to begin.[4] When it's time to touch him, you may **begin with the "outer" parts** of his body first (e.g., counting fingers and toes) and then move centrally towards the trunk.[4] Another approach is to use one of your instruments (e.g., your stethoscope) to intervene between his body and yours, before you actually touch him. (You have to introduce him to the stethoscope first. Try pretending it's a telephone. Place it in your ears. Listen to his knee and say: "hello, hello, anybody there?" . . . David, are you in there?") If he allows it, you can gradually move towards his chest. If he pushes the stethoscope away, don't fight it initially, make a game of bringing it towards him and back again (listening whenever you can). Keep talking, or making interesting sounds. Keep handing him things (including your instruments) to keep him interested and distracted. Remember, the order isn't important. Review the broad outlines of the exam in your mind. Defer ears, posterior pharynx, and the recumbent aspects until the end. Each time you examine a resistant toddler, try out different "games."[1] You'll find out what you're best at. You'll also find out what works best for different situations. You may even need to get down on the floor. **Don't worry about what you look like.** Just concentrate on how well you're doing with your patient. The details of the toddler exam will be reviewed below, in a somewhat traditional order. This is to serve as a memory aid, so when you are trying to remember what you've left out, it will be easier for you.

A few words about the older toddler: your expertise will still be required, but the payoff generally comes easier! Two's may be as difficult to get close to as David was. The two-year-old is terribly anxious about separation, but you know how to handle that! If he is willing to leave his mom, your biggest problem may be trying to "catch" him. Many "two's" are always on the go. He will climb all over the examining room. He will turn on the water in your sink. He will pull his mommy's pocketbook apart. He will love a beeper and enjoy playing with blocks. He will be interested in everything. Use his curiosity to your advantage and pretend with him. When it's time for the exam, he may not leave mom's lap any faster than David did. But he will understand more, so

your dialogue with him will be more productive in enhancing rapport.

Three's and four's are delightful! Some are very outgoing and unafraid as long as they know mom isn't going anywhere, and as long as they know what you're going to do before you do it. Some are very shy and need lots of "warming up" time. Memories of previous experiences at the doctor are likely to impact on the initial interaction. Sometimes this is to your advantage and sometimes it isn't. They have tremendous language and cognitive abilities, which you can use to your advantage. They love being treated as a "big boy or big girl"[1] You can talk to them in simple adult language.[1] They will usually enjoy talking about "school," Sesame Street, and fun things. You can show them your instruments and demonstrate their use. Ask for help in placing your stethoscope on his chest. Make a big show of warming the diaphragm up with your hands, while explaining what you are doing. Ask him to feel the diaphragm and tell you if it's warm enough to place on his chest.[4] If he still looks worried, demonstrate on the parent, older sibling, or doll. If feasible, allow choices. For example, ask him if he would prefer to be examined on the examining table or in his parent's lap. Alternatively, tell him to hop up on the examining table, but ask him where on the chest you should listen to first.[4]

The older toddler may have acquired a fear of bodily harm. Reassurance: verbally ("you don't need any shots today"—if that's true), and physically (slow gentle touch, using demonstration) may help you in this age group. This is also the age at which the true foundations of the future, mature, "doctor-patient" relationship arise. This begins when the clinician offers choices during the exam and continues by involving the patient in conversation about his signs, symptoms, or health care. These actions set the tone for future clinical encounters in which he will be expected to take an increasingly active role. By establishing this pattern of involvement early on, the child may feel more "in control" during his visits and thus more in control about his health in general.[4]

Let's review the details of the toddler exam, keeping in mind that this may be performed as a "lap" exam or a table exam. The "order" resembles the more traditional "head-to-toe" order as the patient nears the older end of the spectrum, and will vary tremendously at the younger end. Ask mom to undress the younger and more wary toddler. Sometimes it's best to have her "strip" him down to the diaper all at once, if he's not too resisting. If the older is hesitant, begin with the parts of the exam that don't require undressing: (e.g., arms, hands, face, development, etc.). Then, either mom or patient can remove one piece of clothing at a time (e.g., sometimes it's necessary to start with the shoes). Sometimes, you will only be allowed to expose one part of the body at a time and be required to replace that item before removing a second one. Be flexible and patient. It will pay off in the end. Continue to include **parents** in your **observations.** Estimating the "goodness of fit" between child and parents includes listening and watching both verbal and nonverbal interactions.

Skin

Observe color and turgor. Note and describe rashes and birthmarks (measure and record size of individual lesions). Some pigmented lesions deserve special mention: cafe-au-lait spots, depigmented spots, and nevocellular nevi. **Cafe-au-lait spots** (Figure 4.1) are well circumscribed, coffee-tan macules. Many normal individuals have one or two small cafe-au-lait spots. Some normal individuals have a large spot or a number of spots. However, if a prepubertal child has 6 or more cafe-au-lait spots, especially if these are larger than ½ cm. in diameter (in the longest axis), you ought to think seriously about the possibility of the diagnosis of the neurocutaneous disorder neurofibromatosis.[5]

Depigmented spots (see Figure 4.2) are flat spots which have less color than the surrounding skin. These, like cafe-au-lait spots are found in many normal individuals. Unfortunately, sometimes a depigmented spot may also be the first sign of another neurocutaneous disorder: tuberous sclerosis. In this disease, the classical shape for the depigmented spot is that of an ash leaf (Figure 4.2). Neurocutaneous diseases have other skin and systemic manifestations which you may read about in a pediatric text. We reviewed cafe-au-lait spots and depigmented spots in particular, because they aren't unusual findings in normal children. In children affected with a neurocutaneous disorder, the cutaneous pigmentary lesions may be the first manifestation of the disease.

The **nevocellular nevus** (Figure 4.3) is a pigmented lesion with cells in the dermis, epidermis, or both. If you find a pigmented

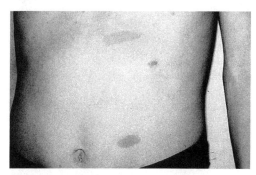

Figure 4.1. Cafe-au-lait spots. Photo courtesy of Stanley F. Glazer, M.D.

Figure 4.2. Ash leaf shaped hypopigmented macule. Reproduced with permission. Hurwitz S. Clinical pediatric dermatology. Philadelphia: W.B. Saunders, 1981:416. Photo courtesy of Sidney Hurwitz, M.D.

growth, ask if the child was born with it. Small congenital nevocellular nevi are usually round or oval in shape and may be found in association with hair follicles. A giant congenital nevocellular nevus which is larger than 10 cm. in length, carries an increased risk for malignant transformation to malignant melanoma. There is less agreement about the smaller lesions, but many dermatologists believe there is increased risk in individuals with these, too. Many pediatricians obtain a consultation whenever a **congenital nevocellular nevus** is found.

During the toddler years, **strawberry hemangiomas** involute. This is gratifying to the practitioner who had to persuade worried, skeptical parents not to intervene during infancy.

Atopic dermatitis (**eczema**) continues to affect children during their toddler years. The dry skin and excoriations may involve any portion of the skin, but from age 2 until adolescence, the rash predominates in the antecubital and popliteal fossae (Figure 4.5).

Discussion of many of the acquired childhood rashes and exanthems is beyond the scope of this book. However, two of these are so common, particularly in toddlers, that deserve mention: impetigo and varicella.

Impetigo (Figure 4.6) is the most common skin infection in children. There are really two types of impetigo which are important to recognize: traditional impetigo

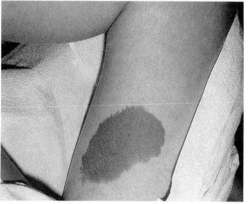

Figure 4.3. Congenital pigmented nevus. Photo courtesy of Stanley F. Glazer, M.D.

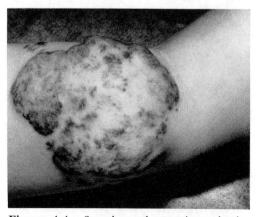

Figure 4.4. Strawberry hemangioma beginning to involute. Photo courtesy of Stanley F. Glazer, M.D.

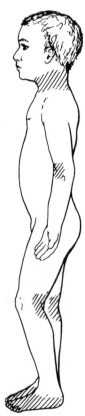

Figure 4.5. Distribution of atopic dermatitis in toddlers and young children: antecubital and popliteal fossae (flexor surfaces). Reproduced with permission. Fleisher GR, Ludwig S., eds. Textbook of pediatric emergency medicine. 2nd ed. Baltimore: Williams & Wilkins, 1988:773.

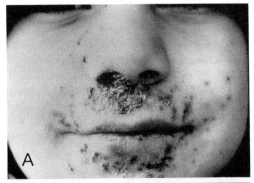

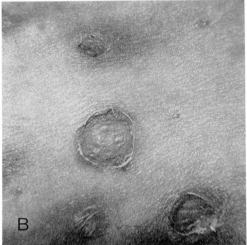

Figure 4.6A. Traditional impetigo. Photograph courtesy of Henry M. Feder, Jr., M.D.
Figure 4.6B. Bullous impetigo. Photograph courtesy of Henry M. Feder, Jr., M.D.

and bullous impetigo. The classic lesion of **traditional impetigo** is a honey colored crust. This lesion begins as a papule and transforms into a vesicle which transforms into a pustule which acquires a honey-colored crust. These lesions are often found at the sight of breaks in the skin. These spread easily and superficially and are contagious. These are not painful, but may be itchy. The causative agent is group A beta hemolytic streptococcus; *Staphylococcus aureus* may be found in conjunction with the strep.[6]

Bullous impetigo (Figure 4.6) is caused by *Staphylococcus aureus*. The primary lesion is a bulla, which is larger than the crust of traditional impetigo. The fluid within the bullae is initially clear and then becomes cloudy. The lesions rupture and leave behind a thin rim of scale. These lesions spread superficially.[6]

If you learn to identify only one childhood exanthem, it should be **varicella** (chickenpox). Most children with this infection are not seen by physicians. This is because the diagnosis is usually made by parents, and children aren't usually sick enough to see the doctor. The exanthem of varicella begins as papules which rapidly transform into the classic lesions which are vesicles on a red base. The fluid in these vesicles rapidly becomes cloudy, after which the vesicles rupture and scab over. Lesions erupt in crops, usually in cycles over the first three or four days, beginning centrally and spreading peripherally, eventually involving not only the trunk, but also the face, scalp, and the extremities. Typically, by the time the disease is well-established, a child is covered with lesions in a variety of stages from papules to vesicles to crusts. Mucous membrane involvement may be present; mouth vesicles rapidly transform into shallow ulcers. Systemic manifestations and numbers of lesions vary tremendously. Some children do not seem ill and have very few lesions; others have high fever for three to five days and are covered from head to toe with cutaneous lesions.

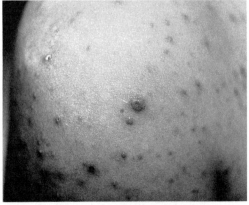

Figure 4.7. Varicella. Photograph courtesy of Henry M. Feder, Jr., M.D.

Head

Assess the head for general appearance: apparent size and marked asymmetries. Feel for prominences (lumps or bumps). If the anterior fontanelle is still open, measure its size.

❓ **By now you can probably predict what I'm going to ask you: At what age should the anterior fontanelle close? Good. Most close by eighteen months; a few normals will remain slightly patent until age 2. During the process of closure, you may feel a firmness before definite "bonyness" within the fontanelle.**

Hair

The quantity, texture and pattern of hair should be noted (include the eyebrows). We mentioned previously that abnormalities of hair may be clues to systemic disease or syndromes. Eyebrows may have the same significance. Eyebrows that meet in the middle (called: synophrys) may be normal or a clue to a syndrome (i.e., Cornelia de Lange syndrome is associated with mental retardation, hirsutism, short stature, and malformations of hands and feet).

Face

Before inspecting individual structures, always obtain an overall impression, Does the child appear bright and alert?, or is there something dull and disinterested about his or her appearance? There may not be anything specific about your observations at this point. You will need to zero in on the individual parts of the exam for more clues. It's just a good habit to get into.

Eyes

Assess shape, size, and symmetry by examining the whole eye and then the individual components as we've discussed in the previous chapters. Note pupillary size, equality, reaction to light and accommodation. Check for a sign of anemia. (Remember how to do this?)

Evaluation of visual acuity in young toddlers is done subjectively, by asking for parental report and by observing toddlers follow or reach for objects placed in all directions in front of them. By age 3 to 4 some toddlers can cooperate for a more formal **vision screen.** In most offices, the nurse will perform the screening before a child is seen for child health maintenance or if there is a history of trauma or visual complaint. If the child you are about to examine is being "screened," go over and watch this being done. You will see how this is performed, but it is also an opportunity to get acquainted with your patient outside of the more formal setting of the examining room. One recommended screening instrument is the Snellen test of distant visual acuity. This chart is placed at eye level at a standardized distance (usually 20 feet) from the child. In preschool and early elementary grade age children, there are several charts such as the tumbling "E" which replace the standard letters on the chart. Each eye should be evaluated separately. While testing one eye, the opposite one should be open but vision occluded. An easy way to accomplish this is to have the child hold an opaque cup over it. In the tumbling "E" test, the child answers by indicating which way the open legs of the "E" are pointing. Some offices use a binocular machine such as Titmus instrument, which incorporates tests for visual acuity, hyperopia, and muscle balance. Children before their fifth birthday should read the 20/40 line. A two-line difference of visual acuity between the eyes, even in the passing range should be evaluated further.[7] These children are at risk for amblyopia.

Back in the examining room, evaluate the toddler for eye muscle imbalance. Check for corneal light reflection symmetry, observe the eyes through range of motion, and perform the alternate cover test. Ask the parents if they've observed any squint, eye crossing, or "lazy" eye.

Practice looking at the fundus. Mom can help you out by holding up an object for the toddler to focus on. Avoid touching the eyes while you look. It will only disturb the toddler and make your exam more difficult. Most of the time, you will get a fleeting glance at the optic disc and the vessels. At this point you ought to aim for familiarizing yourself with the normal appearance of the disc, vessels, and background, including the macula.

Visual field testing isn't part of a standard pediatric examination unless a detailed neurologic or ophthalmologic exam is required. If you need to do this, have the toddler sit on the floor facing a parent who visually distracts him by playing in front of him. Stand behind the child and bring an attractive object from behind him into each of the four quadrants of his field of vision. When he turns his head towards the object, then you know he has seen it. This is a very "gross" test of visual fields.

Ears

Inspect the external ear. Don't forget to look and feel behind the ear. What may be hidden back there are such findings as: mastoid prominence tenderness (seen in mastoiditis), enlarged postauricular nodes (seen with scalp inflammations, childhood exanthems) and rashes (seen in eczema and seborrhea). Children with a basilar skull fracture may have ecchymoses behind the ear (this is called a **Battle's sign**).

Evaluation of hearing (like vision) in young toddlers is performed subjectively, by asking for parental report and by observing the youngster's response to noises made beyond his line of sight. By age 4 some toddlers can cooperate for a more **formal hearing screen.** This is performed using an audiometer (another procedure you will want to observe). If a child fails an audiometric screening (e.g., inability to respond to sounds of 1,000 Hz or 2,000 Hz at 20 dB or 4,000 Hz at 25 dB in either ear) and cooperation has been judged adequate by the examiner, or if parents express concerns about hearing, or if language is significantly impaired or delayed, referral for formal audiologic evaluation is necessary. In a young toddler, defer otoscopic examination till the end of the exam.

Nose

Check for patency and drainage. Examine the mucosa, turbinates, and septum. Unilateral nasal drainage (often green and foul smelling) or swelling, is ultimately encountered by anyone who examines lots of toddlers. The most common cause is a **foreign body** which is usually a wad of tissue, a food remnant, or a bead. If you are lucky, you will be able to spot it way up there inside the nose. Most can be retrieved with a forceps (don't attempt it without help).

Mouth

Inspect the anterior surfaces of the mouth. Toddlers like to have their teeth "counted" (this may afford you an opportunity to inspect all of the mouth!—but if not, don't push it at this point). By age 2 to 2½ most will have a full complement of 20 primary teeth (upper and lower: central incisors, lateral incisors, cuspids, first and second molars). **Milk bottle caries** (or BBTD = Baby bottle tooth decay) are caused by prolonged, usually nighttime contact with a sugar-containing liquid (e.g., from taking a bottle of milk or juice to bed, or breastfeeding all night long). These appear as brown to black discolorations and holes on the central maxillary incisors (the lower incisors are not involved). Involved maxillary anterior teeth and normal mandibular anterior teeth are pathognomonic of BBTD. If severe, all of the upper teeth may be involved (Figure 4.8).

Inspect general oral hygiene. Placques on teeth and generalized erythema or friability of gingivae probably reflect poor oral hygiene. Three-year-olds should have a dental physical exam. In addition, any child with colored stains on teeth (even those with orange-pumpkin colored stains caused by food and plaque) should have a dental check up. The dentist will check for malocclusion, caries, abnormal eruptions, early periodon-

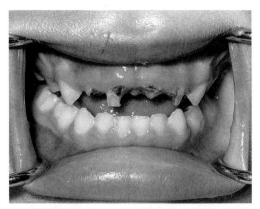

Figure 4.8.   Milk bottle caries.

tal disease and other individual teeth abnormalities. In some communities where there are pediatric dentists, children may be encouraged to go for a preliminary visit even earlier.

By now, you've had ample opportunity to sample your patient's speech. Language development, like all other areas of development may make bumpy or smooth progress. **Listen to both the content and clarity of speech.** If you're not able to achieve cooperation, ask the parents for their observations. By age two, the toddler should be able to make his wants known by using his voice, use at least several words routinely and point correctly to objects such as head or shoe. By age three, he should make two or three word sentences, use "me" or "you" appropriately and respond to simple commands. By age four, the child should be able to correctly give his first and last name, discuss aspects of his daily life, and use plurals and past tenses.[8]

By age three, a child's speech should be relatively easy to understand. However, certain types of **articulation errors** (such as **substituting** "w" for "r" in rabbit, or "d" for "th" in that) are normal in the toddler age group. A two-year-old's speech should be understood approximately fifty percent of the time. Four-year-olds should be understood most of the time. Another clarity issue involves **repetition of sounds or words (stuttering) or hesitations.** These are called **"disfluencies"** and are a **normal** process occurring a year or two after the onset of

speech development. These are not considered **pathologic** or **"dysfluencies"** unless they persist for many months or years and interfere with communication (e.g., involve many syllables or words and evoke tension in the child). Children who fail to communicate within the expected range of normal may need to be evaluated in more detail.[8] This might involve a full physical exam, an audiologic exam, and a referral to a speech and language expert.

Unless the toddler voluntarily opens his mouth, defer examination of the pharynx until the end of the exam.

Neck

Inspect for bulges (e.g., significantly enlarged lymph nodes), head tilts, and thyromegaly. The thyroid gland should not be visible. If it is, then it is enlarged. After inspection, palpate the neck all around. The **small, mobile, soft,** nontender lymph nodes in healthy children, most commonly found high up in the anterior or posterior cervical triangles, at the occiput and angle of the jaw, are called **"shotty."** Sometimes these are visible bumps of great concern to parents. Their characteristic qualities and location are reassuringly normal. If lymph nodes are enlarged, tender, hard, or numerous they should be counted, measured, and described. Anterior cervical adenopathy (an increased number and/or size of nodes above normal) accompanies upper respiratory infections and inflammation of the anterior portions of the mouth. Posterior cervical adenopathy accompanies otitis media, some viral infections, and scalp irritations. All of these may take many weeks to resolve. There are many "typical" patterns of lymph node enlargement which are consistent with the numerous infections and rashes of childhood. Your goal right now should be to learn what "shotty" nodes feel like and what their usual distribution is. When you begin to examine children with adenopathy, become a detective: locate and describe enlarged nodes, figure out what area they drain, and attempt to uncover the most likely etiology.

Evaluate **range of motion.** How do you accomplish this in a patient too young to follow directions? Hold aloft an attractive object and move it in all directions, while observing the patient's head movement.

When you encounter a child in whom meningeal irritation (e.g., from meningitis) is a possibility, you will need to know how to assess for **nuchal rigidity** (stiff neck in the anterior-posterior direction). There are other reasons for a stiff neck besides meningitis (e.g., cervical spine abnormalities, severe pharyngitis—remember the child mentioned previously who had a peritonsillar abscess?), and not all children with meningitis have nuchal rigidity. But if nuchal rigidity is present, it's very important to know about it. This procedure should only be attempted in the child who normally has excellent head control (that's why we didn't discuss this in the infant chapter). Practice assessment for nuchal rigidity in healthy toddlers until you are comfortable with the maneuver and the expected results. Then when you encounter an ill, less cooperative child you will be prepared to identify deviations from normal. At this point in the exam, it's likely that the toddler is still sitting up. Rather than lay him down now, wait until he is supine to do this. The evaluation is included in this space merely for completeness sake:

To evaluate for **nuchal rigidity** (Figure 4.9), have the toddler lie supine on the examining table. Cradle the back of his head in your hands and gently flex the head at the neck until his chin touches his chest. Assess the degree of resistance of this maneuver. When meningeal irritation is present, it will be **very** difficult to flex the neck. Even healthy children may resist and cry but will allow flexion. It's important to do this slowly and gently, in a non-crying child if at all possible. Distraction with your voice or eyes may help. If this maneuver causes him to flex his knees up off the table, this is called a **Brudzinski sign** and is also a sign of meningeal irritation. Third, while he's su-

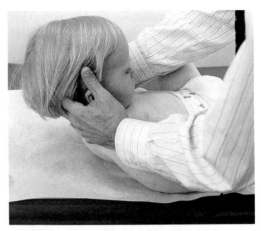

Figure 4.9.   Testing for nuchal rigidity.

pine, if you flex his thigh at the hip 90° and then cannot straighten out the leg at the knees, this is called a **Kernig sign.** A Kernig sign is associated with meningeal irritation and hamstring spasm.

Finally, (back to the child who is still sitting up), a child with meningeal irritation will not be able or willing to look down onto his chest no matter what tricks you attempt. A child who doesn't really have a stiff neck, but simply doesn't want to be touched can be tricked into looking down at his chest. If you say, "Hey, you have a spot on your shirt," the child with meningismus will not look down, but the child without it, will.

Thorax and Upper Extremities

Inspect clavicles, thorax, and upper extremities. Palpate along and above clavicles, and in the axillae. Palpate pulses. Examine the upper extremities, including the hands and fingers. Range of motion, bulk, tone and strength of the upper extremities should be assessed in addition to attending to the skin and nails. Older toddlers will cooperate for **assessment of grip strength** by squeezing your fingers "hard," while younger ones will demonstrate their strength by actively pushing you away! In addition, the older toddler may "help" you count their fingers. This maneuver can supply you with information about their development as well as their speech.

If you are suspicious about **anemia,** inspect the palm creases. These should be flesh or pink colored. If the creases look slightly paler than the rest of the skin of the palm, suspect anemia.

Cardiorespiratory

Inspect the precordium, palpate the precordium and the PMI. The PMI in the toddler is located in approximately the same position as in the infant.

❓ What is the location of the PMI in the infant? . . . Right! It's in the 4th intercostal space, just to the left of the midclavicular line. Feel for thrills, heaves, or lifts.

Auscultate the heart over the precordium, axillae, neck, and back using both the bell and the diaphragm. Getting a "quiet" exam from a young toddler (and a recumbent one too) isn't easy. This is where help from distracting toys and mom is required. (As mentioned in the previous chapter, if your patient is both healthy and unlikely to cooperate, seize the moment and listen to the heart, instead of palpating the precordium). Hopefully, you've allowed adequate time for the toddler to feel and play with your stethoscope before attempting to put the "warmed" head onto his chest. You may have to break this exam up into several parts during the course of your encounter to get a decent listen. The older toddler may do very well during cardiac auscultation.

Auscultate for rate and rhythm, then listen to each sound individually. Finally, listen for murmurs and any other adventitious sounds such as clicks or rubs (describing: location, radiation, intensity, duration, and change with position). The cooperative older toddler will probably not mind having you listen in both the upright and recumbent positions. With the less cooperative child, you should listen first in the upright position and save the recumbent component until you examine the abdomen.

Most childhood **innocent murmurs** are first heard in the three- or four-year-old. The explanation for this phenomenon may have two components: this is the first time, after the neonatal period, that one is able to reliably secure a cooperative "quiet" patient. In addition, the less rounded and less padded chest of the older toddler may make it easier to hear the heart sounds. There are three innocent murmurs of childhood that are often first heard in this age group: Still's murmur, Venous hum, and Carotid bruit.

❓ What are the characteristics of innocent murmurs we listed earlier? Yes: Innocent murmurs are usually of low intensity which often varies with repositioning the patient up or down (not louder than a grade 3/6). They do not have a harsh or grating quality. They do not radiate widely. They are never associated with other adventitious sounds (such as clicks) or other features of abnormal cardiovascular exams (such as heaves or cyanosis). Except for the continuous venous hum, they are never found in diastole. The systolic component of innocent murmurs are also *never* regurgitant. That is, they never begin with S1, they always begin *after* S1.

The **Still's murmur** is a low pitched systolic ejection murmur with a musical or vibratory quality (as distinguished from a pathologic harsh or grating sound). It's best heard halfway between the lower left sternal border and the apex, with increased intensity in the supine position. It will sound louder with fever or exercise.

The **Venous hum** is a continuous (heard in systole and diastole) murmur heard best on the right side of the chest at the level of the clavicles (may also be heard at the left infraclavicular area). It may be obliterated or modified by turning the patient's head away from the side of the murmur or compressing the internal jugular vein on the side of the murmur. It disappears in the supine position. The sounds arise from blood flow through the great veins in the neck.

The **Carotid bruit** is a systolic ejection murmur (not louder than a grade 3/6) that is heard over the carotids. It diminishes as the auscultation approaches the aortic or pulmonic areas (which distinguishes it from valvular murmurs).

First work on learning these innocent murmurs. Once you've learned to identify them, you will see how different most pathologic ones sound.

Starting at age 3, (unless there are concerns about hypertension earlier) yearly blood pressure measurements should be performed at child health maintenance visits. The directions for this are found in the measurements section. An accurate reading can only be obtained from a calm and cooperative patient. You may choose to defer this until the end of the exam.

Listen over the anterior and posterior lung fields. Count respiratory rate and observe for increased respiratory effort. Listen for adequacy of aeration and for adventitious sounds. When you begin your lung exam with a cooperative 3- or 4-year-old (especially one who has been "prepared" for the visit by his parents) he sometimes tries to "help" you by taking a big breath in and then holding it. It's best not to give him directions before you begin. Just listen to quiet breathing. If you have difficulty hearing end expiratory sounds (these are the most difficult to hear—but may be the most important): gently compress the chest between your examining hand (e.g., the one holding the stethoscope on the back) and your other hand placed on the opposite side of the chest (e.g., in the front) or vice versa (Figure 4.10). This accentuates expiration and makes end expiratory sounds (like wheezes) easier to hear.

Previously we've discussed the "merits" of listening to the crying toddler: listening in inspiration will be a breeze. To hear expiration, you will have to wait till he calms down.

In the previous chapter, you learned a method to distinguish "nose" sounds from the crackles and wheezes coming from the lungs. Stridor is another respiratory sound which you may encounter. This is a harsh sound heard with inspiration. It originates

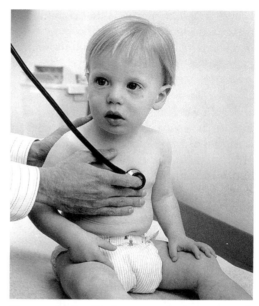

Figure 4.10. During auscultation, chest is compressed with free hand to accentuate expiratory sounds.

from the larynx and/or trachea when there is obstruction present in either. You only need to hear stridor once. After that you will never forget it. Each time you encounter a child with noisy breathing, ask yourself: Where are the sounds coming from? Do the sounds come from the nose, larynx/trachea, or lungs? If you can answer this question, you're more than half way to a diagnosis.

Infants and toddlers may also contract pneumonia. Small children with pneumonia may have signs of respiratory distress, crackles, or wheezes. They may also have signs of a generalized infection without any definite pulmonary findings. Sometimes, even though they seem to be working hard to breathe, you will not hear clearly identifiable adventitious sounds. This is particularly true in the younger child, the crying child, or the child with decreased air entry.

Abdomen

As toddlers grow, they gradually slim out, but the "belly" is often the last to go until abdominal musculature strengthens. Parents frequently ask about their toddler's "pot belly." The lumbar lordosis of childhood makes the abdomen further appear to "stick out." Before you begin your abdominal exam, make sure your hands and stethoscope are warm. Most toddlers are quite "ticklish" and a cold hand or instrument on their abdomen won't make your exam any easier. The other problem you will encounter is getting the young toddler to lie down. The older toddler, by this point in the exam, has hopefully learned to trust you. If you can't coax the two-year-old into the recumbent position (even in his mom's lap) you may have to do this exam while he is sitting or standing. The quality of your exam won't be as good, but it's better than nothing. Fortunately, finding unexpected intrabdominal pathology in this age group is extremely rare.

If you are successful in exposing the abdomen for the exam, follow inspection with auscultation for bowel sounds. If your patient resists you, have him "hold" the stethoscope on his abdomen (if you need to exert more pressure, push down on his fingers gently). See if you can guess what he "had for lunch." Conversations like this are useful distractors.

Begin palpation superficially and increase pressure gradually. Feel for the liver edge (1 to 2 cm. below the right costal margin) and spleen tip (if slightly enlarged, may be slightly palpable in the older infant at the left costal margin). Feel for masses. Note tenseness and tenderness. The abdomen should be soft and nontender, but the toddler is so wiggly during this exam, he may jump and squirm whenever he is touched. A helpful maneuver (besides distraction either with a toy or conversation) is to again ask for "help" from your older toddler patient. If he is supine, have him flex his legs at the hips and knees so the soles of his feet grip the surface of the table. Then ask him to place his hand (or hands) on top of yours, and request that **he "do the pushing."** The older toddler will enjoy participating in the exam; in addition, the work of pushing down on your hands often distracts him enough to relax his abdomen (see Figure 4.11).

If abdominal pain is a complaint, you may ask an older toddler to point to "where it hurts." However, don't expect much from the answer. The younger the child, the more difficulty he will have in localizing the site of abdominal pain. Not infrequently, a cooperative child will point to the umbilicus. That may mean that it hurts there, but it may also reflect referred pain from somewhere else. Unfortunately, the answer, while an honest one, may also reflect the child's true inability to localize the origin of abdominal pain. You will not necessarily be able to figure out which of those factors are operating. If a toddler does tell you where it hurts, begin palpation away from that area and return to it after having palpated the rest of the abdomen. In a cooperative patient with true localized tenderness, the tenderness will be reproducible. While you are palpating, see if you can engage the patient in a conversation, as true tenderness may make the patient grimace or interrupt an answer in midsentence. Rebound tenderness, like true

Figure 4.11. Maneuver to relax the abdomen. Ask the patient to "help do the pushing."

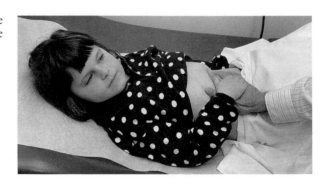

tenderness, is also more difficult to elicit accurately in young children. But it may be there. If your patient is suspected of having an acute abdomen, don't forget to attempt to elicit rebound too (in an area away from the site of maximal tenderness, press in deeply, then rapidly remove your fingers). You may also elicit rebound tenderness by holding the pelvis and gently shaking the abdomen side to side.

If you note the presence of an umbilical hernia, measure it and feel for bowel contents within it. These should be easily reducible.

The "mass" felt most often in toddlers, is fecal matter in the colon. This may feel like hard round balls in the left lower quadrant (in which case they will be freely mobile). Sometimes you can even outline a large sausage-shaped mass filling the entire descending colon.

Percussion of the abdomen in well children isn't routine. If you suspect intraabdominal pathology (e.g., organomegaly, mass, or ascites) then percuss in the manner of the adult exam.

Genitalia

Getting the diaper down off of a toddler is no easy task. Ask mom to assist you. Tell the older toddler that you are going to "take a peek" at her bottom to check to see that everything looks o.k. Tell her that it won't hurt. (Don't ask permission. She'll say no.) Just proceed matter of factly down from the abdomen and continue without missing a beat.

Inspect the genitalia and the anus carefully. Palpate the inguinal regions and femoral pulse.

Female: Inspect the genitalia by separating the labia. Not infrequently, toddler girls develop mild vaginal itching and/or discharge associated with nonspecific irritation. The vagina and perineum may appear red and slightly swollen, and a watery vaginal discharge may be visible. Genital itching and irritation may also accompany pinworm infestation of the gastrointestinal tract. Thin thread-like worms may be visible around the anus, but these are usually not visible except in the early morning. Unfortunately, vaginal discharge may also be a sign of a sexually transmitted disease and sexual abuse. Whenever you are examining a child who has genital complaints, you must consider the possibility of sexual abuse. In any case, always "tune into" genital tears, bruises, or scars, or enlargement of the introitus. Unfortunately, the physical exam is often normal, even with documented abuse. Remember, too, that the presence of vaginal or perianal warts must raise the suspicion of abuse.

Another etiology for vaginal discharge is a foreign body. The foreign body is usually a wad of facial tissue or toilet tissue. Occasionally, it might even be a small toy. Toddlers put foreign bodies into **every** orifice. Careful, gentle inspection may reveal the secret.

Male: Examine the penis. Retract the foreskin gently. Be age three, ninety percent of males will have a fully retractable foreskin. Palpate the scrotum and testicles (and milk them into the scrotum if necessary). (Occasionally, an undescended testicle may go unnoticed until the toddler age group: be sure that you palpate **both** testicles). Keep in mind also that inguinal hernias may appear at any age.

Back

If your patient is a toddler who is "all over the place" during your encounter, you will have ample opportunity to examine his back, especially when he turns away from you and clutches desperately at his mom (use **every** opportunity presented to you to **observe**). Alternatively, you may examine the back after the recumbent portion of the exam. Remember to look at the posterior neck and then run your eyes down the length of the spine observing for straightness and symmetry of lateral structures such as the shoulders, scapulae, and iliac crests. Once a toddler's balance is stable enough, you should perform this exam while his feet are touching side by side. Palpate the spine for lesions or tenderness. While he's ambulating, make sure that he doesn't splint movement in any particular direction. Curvature of the spine (scoliosis) isn't a common problem in normal children prior to the late school or preadolescent period. If there is an apparent curvature, or range of motion is limited, or lateral landmarks aren't symmetric, refer to the next chapter for details about scoliosis assessment. The normal toddler, when viewed from the side, has an **exaggerated lower lumbar lordosis** (Figure 4.12). This forward curvature of the spine is partly responsible for the toddler "pot" belly. In school-age children, the curve becomes less prominent.

Lower Extremities

Before you have your toddler stand and walk, inspect the lower extremities and put them through a range of motion. Strength and tone may be assessed simultaneously. You're now an expert on separating out the various parts of the lower extremities: hips, thighs, knees, legs, and feet.

Watch him stand and walk. Wait . . . what

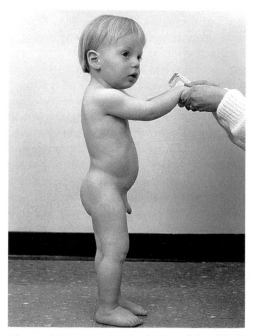

Figure 4.12. Lumbar lordosis and "pot" belly of the toddler.

do you do if he won't walk, but rather clings to his mom's leg? . . . Quickly pick him up, walk across the room, and put him down. He will walk or run right back to his mom. . . .

Note asymmetries and limitations of movement. The wide base of the novice comes together during the later toddler years. The **feet will appear flat.** This is usually related to the presence of fat pads which obscure the longitudinal arch of the foot. Some new walkers **walk on their toes** initially and within months, gradually lose the habit. Some have a family history of toe walking without any underlying pathology. Persistence of toe walking requires a very thorough neuromuscular exam, as children with spastic diplegia or muscular dystrophy may also demonstrate toe walking.

Before two years of age it is common for a child to be mildly bowlegged. From age 3 to 5 years, it is common for a child to be mildly knockkneed. In most instances, there is a spontaneous correction to a straight-legged stance by age 7 or 8. Severe cases which do not improve require orthopedic attention.

In order to answer the most common question from parents about gait: ("Why do his feet turn in?") you need to have one more orthopedic tool: estimating the angle of gait. The **angle of gait** is the "angle between the axis of the foot and the line of progression."[9] Most children and adults walk with their feet pointed outward or externally rotated. During childhood, this angle is usually about 10° from the line of progression. Persistent intoeing or outtoeing more than 30° is abnormal.[10] If your patient intoes more than 30°, it is likely that forces at the hip, along the shaft of the tibia, or at the feet are responsible (Figure 4.13).

❓ **You already know how to examine for the most common causes of intoeing at the feet and along the tibia. What are they? Yes: metatarsus adductus and tibial torsion. You examined the newborn for the former and the older infant for both. If your patient**

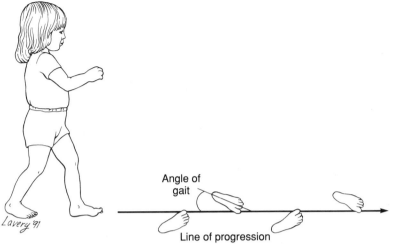

Figure 4.13. Estimating the angle of gait (how much does the child toe in or out). The angle of gait is estimated as the average angle that each step makes with the line of progression. Redrawn with permission: Staheli LT. Torsional deformity. Pediatr Clin North Am, 1977;24:802.

intoes, repeat the diagnostic maneuvers you have learned for each problem.

To round-out your initial course on intoeing, examine for **increased femoral anteversion** (at the hip), which is the most common cause of intoeing. In the normal infant and young child the degree of external rotation of the hip exceeds internal rotation (they are approximately equal in older children). In patients with increased femoral anteversion, the degree of internal rotation is greater than normal (e.g., greater than 70°). How do you figure out what the degree of rotation at the hip is? Have your patient lie belly down on the table. Flex the knees (with the hips in extension) and determine the arc that each leg circumscribes (from the vertical) as it falls by gravity into internal rotation and as it crosses the midline (in the opposite direction) into external rotation (Figure 4.14). This is a little confusing, I know. It is helpful to remember that inward and outward rotation refer to the head of the femur. So when you are allowing the leg to fall outward with gravity, you are really rotating the head of the femur inward (internal rotation), and when you are moving the leg across the midline, you are really rotating the head of the femur outward

(external rotation). If you can move the leg much farther into internal rotation than into external rotation, then you have made a diagnosis of increased femoral anteversion.[10]

Why do children outtoe? The newborn normally outtoes (you just don't realize it, because he isn't walking!). The reason is because intrauterine positioning forces the baby into external rotation at the hip. At birth, the hip is contracted into this position. During the course of the first year to year and a half, crawling and early walking stretch-out this contracture. Once a child is walking well, outtoeing is much less common than intoeing. Now that you are an expert on examining the legs, I bet you can guess two other causes of outtoeing! Yes: femoral retroversion (rare) and external tibial torsion (rare in isolation).[11] You know how to examine for both of these!

Parents may ask you about **tripping.** All children until middle school age trip and fall when they run. Obviously, some trip more than others. You require both history and physical exam to answer parents' question. If, after two years of walking well, a child suddenly begins to fall a lot, this is much more likely to signify a problem than if he has always tripped occasionally. A child with normal gait and a normal neurologic exam

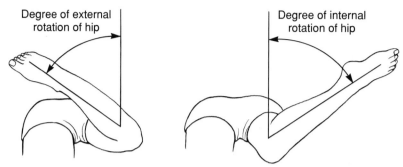

Figure 4.14. Assessment of external and internal rotation at the hip. Redrawn with permission: Staheli LT. Torsional deformity. Pediatr Clin North Am 1977;24:803.

(including balance) who sometimes trips when he runs will probably outgrow this normal developmental phenomenon.

In addition to learning to perform a routine orthopedic assessment on a healthy toddler, you must also be prepared for the not infrequent encounter with a toddler who has a limp or reluctance to walk. Make sure your history includes thorough questions about the possibility of trauma. Even if there is no history of trauma, an injury is still a possibility. A toddler without trauma, who refuses to walk, often has an **irritable hip.** He may have fever. He is usually unable to correctly localize the source of the pain. In fact, even an older child with an irritable hip may point to the thigh or knee as the source of the pain. This is because hip pain is frequently referred to the thigh and the knee. Examine the child in the supine position. Decide whether or not the leg in question is held in a different position than the unaffected one. Determine if there is a difference in the range of motion between the joints of the two lower extremities. Palpate from hip to feet for any tenderness. In addition, palpate the hip joint at the anteromedial thigh immediately distal to the inguinal fold; if there is an inflammatory effusion, there may be signs of swelling and tenderness. The most common cause of an irritable hip in a toddler is toxic synovitis of the hip, which is an inflammation of the hip joint of unknown etiology. As with any hip irritation, there is reduced range of motion at the hip, with the limb held in partial hip

flexion, abduction, and external rotation. Full passive internal rotation is difficult to achieve. The differential diagnosis includes infectious, arthritic, metabolic and posttraumatic problems. X-rays, blood work, and analysis and culture of aspirated joint fluid may be required to rule-out some of these other serious causes. Right now, you should concentrate on learning to identify the site which is the source of the pain.

Neurologic and Development

Mentally review these exams and fill in what you've left out. Earlier in the encounter, you may have chosen to play with your patient in order to put him at ease. If play included such tasks as drawing with crayons or perusing a picture book and discussing its contents, you probably have a good idea about his developmental milestones in those areas. With the older more cooperative toddler, much of the neurologic exam will begin to resemble what you have been taught in adults.

General Appearance and Mental Status. Review your observations of state, mood, cognitive skills and language. Specific developmental tasks are found under the "developmental milestones" section of the appropriate history flow sheet. Also included under general appearance are growth parameters, skin, dysmorphic features, head, and spine.

Cranial Nerves. Assess as completely as possible (II–XII). Review the maneuvers you've already performed, (e.g., extraocular movements that require intact functioning of **III, IV,** and **VI**) and fill in what's been left out. Just as a reminder: Assessment of **II** includes estimate of visual acuity, fundus exam (older toddler may be able to cooperate), and gross estimation of visual fields. Assessment of **III, IV, and VI** includes estimate of pupil size, observation of pupillary reaction to light and accommodation, and extraocular muscle coordination. Assessment of **V** includes inspection and palpation for symmetry of the masseter and temporal muscles with a clenched jaw, observing for symmetry of upper and lower incisors, observation of equal jaw movement with side to side motion of the jaw and strength in holding on to a tongue stick with teeth opposed. The corneal reflex isn't routinely evaluated in a healthy child, but if necessary may be attempted in the same fashion as in newborns. Assessment of **VII** includes inspecting for facial symmetry during smiling, eye closure, and blowing. Asking the parent about tear function should suffice (you will probably have the chance to make this observation yourself). Assess hearing **VIII,** either subjectively or objectively as described earlier in this chapter. Cranial nerves **IX and X** are assessed by observing palatal and uvula position and movement, an intact gag reflex, and normal phonation. Cranial nerve **XI** which controls the sternocleidomastoid muscle may be assessed by observing a normal head position and the ability to flex the neck and turn the head; the trapezius may be assessed by asking the patient to shrug his shoulders against resistance imposed by the examiner's hands. Demonstrate this. Last, **XII** is assessed by inspection of the tongue for fasciculations (very fine local contractions) and movement of the tongue in all directions (you will have plenty of opportunity to observe this shortly if you use a tongue blade to inspect the posterior pharynx).

Motor. Observe and palpate bulk; you've assessed tone with passive movements of limbs and strength by opposition (you've probably gotten lots of that!). Observe gross motor (looking for asymmetries and weakness) in such movements as: walking, sitting up, getting on and off the examining table or the floor, heel walking, etc. Observe fine motor manipulations of blocks, crayons, figure copying, etc.

Ask your patient to squat down on the floor, then get (or jump) up (you may have to squat down with him to secure his cooperation for this game). A child with muscle weakness in the lower back and pelvic girdle (proximal) (e.g., a child with Duchenne muscular dystrophy) will get off the floor in a characteristic fashion (called a **Gower's** sign). He will be unable to jump right up, but rather will need to "walk" his hands up the front of his lower extremities (bracing against them), until he is upright.

Coordination. You may make these observations while observing gross and fine motor movement as in the previous sections. Arm swing, fluidity of movement, and balance should be observed. The four-year-old should be able to imitate rapid thumb to forefinger opposition.

Station and Gait. Observe your patient standing (we've already described the typical stance of the toddler). By age three or four he should be able to stand erect with feet together and maintain balance with eyes open and closed (a Romberg test). When he walks, observe for asymmetries, limp, foot dragging, toe walking, or ataxia.

Unwanted Movements. Observe for tremors, myoclonus, tics, or other involuntary abnormal movements.

Sensory. Formal evaluation of sensation is usually reserved for those in whom there are special neurologic concerns. A few older toddlers can cooperate for evaluation of spinal sensation involving tests of response to light touch or pin, joint movements, or sensation of tuning fork. Cortical sensation testing may also be difficult, but not impossible, to perform; it may include discriminating objects placed in the hand and/or discriminating simple shapes drawn by the examiner's finger on the body.

Reflexes. Deep tendon reflexes may be assessed in the traditional fashion. It's helpful to have an extra hammer around; offer one to your patient. Show him how to "assess" your reflexes first, demonstrate on his mom. The Babinski sign should be absent. The "primitive" reflexes of the newborn and infant should be absent.

Ears and Pharynx

In the toddler age group, this exam is usually deferred until the latter part of the visit (unless of course, this is a problem visit for an earache). Even under that circumstance, the rest of the general physical exam should be performed first.

The child under two is not only less willing to have his ears examined than the one-year-old, he's also stronger. Rarely, you will encounter an unusually cooperative two-year-old. But most of the time you will not. Therefore, the key here is to plan immobilization carefully before you begin, by giving very specific instructions to your "helper" (usually mom). You may choose to examine him on the table or in mom's lap. The key to my decision usually rests in how well I believe mom will restrain her child. If I'm concerned about her ability to do this, I usually use the examining table (it's easier to restrain children there). Don't think of yourself as the "bad guy" (or woman). The better a child is restrained, the less chance of injury during the exam (injury to the child that is). The ear canal is surprisingly fragile, and contact between a fighting child and an otoscope, all too often results in a bleeding canal!

Some three- or four-year-olds won't cooperate either, but I start by giving them the benefit of the doubt. I give them choices as to where they'd like to sit while being examined. I also ask them which ear they'd like me to look in first. I also use some distraction technique as I look (e.g., I make clicking sounds while I look in the younger child's ear, or I might ask the older toddler if he thinks I'll find any potatoes growing inside).

When you're set, pull up and back on the auricle and peek at the canal as you enter it with the otoscope. Look for signs of inflammation. Remember the foreign bodies we've talked about? Guess where else toddlers put them! If the ear hurts when you pull back on the auricle, then there is probably an otitis externa (swimmer's ear, inflammation of the canal). But, as otitis externa is often associated with submersion of the head during swimming, it is uncommon in this young age group.

Examine the drum for color, landmarks, and visible fluid behind it. When you think you've got an airtight seal, insufflate the rubber bulb and observe the drum for the normal response.

I've previously remarked about the possibility of finding a surprise acute otitis media. Parents have some difficulty believing this finding, when their child has seemed perfectly well (me too!). There are two additional tympanic membrane conditions which are common findings in asymptomatic or healthy-appearing children. The first is **tympanosclerosis** in which there are white plaques in the eardrum. These are usually sequelae of prior infections and are of no consequence unless the entire drum is so scarred that movement with insufflation is inhibited. The second condition is **serous otitis media.** Serous otitis implies the presence of fluid in the middle ear without acute inflammation. Bacteria can sometimes be cultured from this fluid, but it is believed that acute infection is absent. Serous otitis occurs as a sequelae of acute purulent otitis media. It may also occur without a preceding bacterial infection, especially in the presence of an upper respiratory infection. In serous otitis, the eardrum appears dull (less shiny and translucent than normal). The color of the drum is either gray, white, or slightly yellow (but the "angry" red or yellow of acute infection is absent). The landmarks may be partly obscured by fluid. The movement in response to insufflation is reduced or absent. There may be an air-fluid level or bubbles visible behind the drum. Serous otitis media is more difficult to diagnose than acute otitis media, because the findings are more subtle. Recognizing serous otitis will take a lot of practice (so look at as many eardrums as you can!) (Figure 4.15).

If the toddler is crying, shine your flashlight in the mouth and examine the posterior pharynx. If not, and he isn't likely to cooperate, use your tongue blade, applying firm pressure on the tongue (you may gently rotate at the wrist (pronate—supine and so forth) while moving posteriorly until you elicit a gag; then look quickly.

A three- or four-year-old may sometimes be convinced to say "ahh", (or "pant like a doggy"), particularly if you hold off on presenting the tongue blade (sometimes this may avoid needing the stick).

Examine the gums, buccal mucosa, tongue, palate, uvula, tonsils, and posterior pharynx. Look for signs of inflammation, ulcers, and other lesions. If you look carefully, you will see lots of oral ulcers in ill children, the vast majority of which are related to viral infection.

Adenoids aren't visible, but the tonsils are clearly visible and may appear large. Maximal development of the lymphoid system occurs prior to puberty. Tonsils and adenoids are involved in this steady normal growth, and therefore **tonsils will be larger in toddlers than in infants.** Second, be-

Figure 4.15. Serous otitis media. Fleisher GR, Ludwig S., eds. Reproduced with permission. Textbook of pediatric emergency medicine. 2nd ed. Baltimore: Williams & Wilkins, 1988:428.

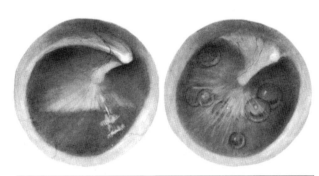

Acute serous ASOM	Chronic serous CSOM
Prominent short process Malleus shortened and retracted Dull	Malleus shortened Air bubbles Dull

cause of the high frequency of upper respiratory infections in toddlers, the involved lymph tissues are often further enlarged by hyperplasia. Tonsil size is commonly described on a grading system of 0–4 with 1 being clearly visible and 4 meaning that tonsils meet or almost meet in the midline (or obstruct at least ¾ of the airway). Crypts in the tonsillar tissue are normal. "Enlarged tonsils," without signs of inflammation, which do not interfere with swallowing or breathing functions are not pathologic. In toddlers, an erythematous pharynx, with or without exudate, is usually caused by a viral infection (under age 4, group A beta hemolytic strep is an unusual pathogen for pharyngitis).

While you are peering into the back of the throat, you may see the epiglottis (often happens with a cooperative older toddler and school age child). This is a normal finding in children. The epiglottis descends to its final lower position (where it is not usually visible) during puberty. During your pediatric experiences you will learn about epiglottitis, a serious bacterial disease of infancy and toddler years. In this disease, the epiglottis is swollen and erythematous (the patient will look very ill and have stridor and air hunger). The normal epiglottis is pink. Look for the epiglottis when you examine cooperative healthy children, so that you become accustomed to its normal color, size, and conformation.

Adenoidal enlargement can be suspected in the presence of "mouth breathing" and "nasal" speech. Direct visualization requires the use of a nasopharyngeal mirror; this is the territory of the Ear, Nose, and Throat specialist.

When your physical exam is completed, compliment your patient on a "job well done." After any further procedures are completed, take your patient to the "sticker box" and let him pick out a reward (or if your patient is too young, bring him something). The examination of the young toddler is probably one of the most exhausting experiences you will have in your pediatric physical diagnosis course or pediatric rotations. However, once you learn some of the special tricks and techniques, it will also be the most satisfying!

THE PROBLEM: "ANOTHER COLD . . . I'M SURE HE HAS SOMETHING WRONG WITH HIM!"

Later in the morning, on that same bright spring day, (when you diagnosed your first otitis media), Ellen hands you another chart. This one belongs to Peter, who is three years old. Ellen says, "He's got a cold. This is about his fifth visit since the fall."

This time, you have his old chart. You sit down for a moment to review it. You see that there are a lot of "problem visits" during the past six months. The diagnoses are most URIs (upper respiratory infections). Peter has also had two episodes of otitis media. At his last health care maintenance visit (two months ago), he had some residual fluid behind his left tympanic membrane (serous otitis). He was scheduled for an "ear check" a week ago, but he was a "no-show" for that appointment. He has had a few visits for minor trauma (a fall off of his tricycle which resulted in a laceration of his arm requiring suturing and a forehead contusion from a fall out of his bed). There are no other significant problem visits and no other infections noted. His past medical history and family history are not out of the ordinary.

When you enter the room, Mrs. Erlin seems to be staring off into space and Peter is looking at a picture book. You introduce yourself. Mrs. Erlin looks exhausted. She explains that Peter has been up for most of the past several nights, unable to sleep "because he can't breathe." She says: "I'm sick and tired of this. You have to give him something to help him!" You explain that you need to find out more about this illness, and then you will examine Peter. (You're feeling more confident about the diagnosis of otitis media. If Peter has it, you'll diagnose it).

You obtain a "history of present illness" and find out that Peter was well until three days ago, when he developed a runny nose and a cough. (Ah ha, you've heard this before!) He has had difficulty breathing through his nose especially at night. Propping him up on a few pillows hasn't helped either his nose or his cough. The mucus from his nose is clear. He has not had a fever. He vomited once last night during a coughing spell. He does not have diarrhea. He does not have ear pain or pain anywhere else. His appetite is only fair, but he is willing to drink apple juice. While you obtain the history from Mrs. Erlin, you can't help but notice that she seems somewhat hostile. Is it because you are a student? You're not sure.

Before you examine Peter, you remember to ask, "Is there anything else about this that's bothering you?" (Good! You remembered hidden agendas!) Mrs. Erlin starts to cry. This really startles you. She explains that she had to put Peter in day care about six months ago, at the time that she and Mr. Erlin separated. They are still separated. Mrs. Erlin had to leave her part-time librarian job (which she enjoyed) and begin a full-time job as a secretary (which she hates) to earn enough money to support herself and Peter. Mr. Erlin sees Peter twice a week, but he doesn't provide child support. Ever since Peter started day care, he's been "sick all the time." She's worried that there's something really wrong with him. She hates to leave him at day care.

Talk about hidden agendas; you hit the jackpot! You decide to gather some more history before you begin your exam. Peter's behavior is usually o.k., except when he's sick. He likes day care and he seems to enjoy playing with the other children. Sometimes he doesn't share too well. He misses his father. His behavior deteriorates just after a visit with his dad.

You also find out that Peter's growth and development has been essentially normal. He "did everything on time" (this is confirmed by his chart). His speech is excellent. He speaks in long sentences, and is easily understood. Mrs. Erlin thinks he hears pretty well (when he wants to). He doesn't snore. He doesn't usually have difficulty breathing.

You take a deep breath to gather your thoughts. There are multiple problems which need to be addressed (this is not exactly a "routine" URI!). You list them mentally:

1. Upper respiratory infection
2. Anything else going on acutely?
3. Mother's concern about a chronic illness or an underlying illness (e.g., something bad?). This concern is aggravated by:
4. Social situation: effects on Peter, effects on Mrs. Erlin (By the way, this information **was** hinted at in the chart. If you'd noticed it before this would have been less of a surprise.)
5. Serous otitis: has this resolved?
6. Missed appointment

You're going to need to address each of these problems. Time to do the physical exam.

Peter is a surprisingly cheerful fellow. He willingly cooperates for an exam. He tells you all about his "school," his friends, and his favorite t.v. shows (Sesame Street and Mr. Rogers). He has an occasional wet sounding cough. He has clear mucus draining at all times from his nose.

His temperature is 99° orally (Ellen used the electronic, nonbreakable thermometer for this). His heart rate is 95. His respiratory rate is 30. His blood pressure is 95/60. His weight is 32 pounds (the same as it was at his health care maintenance visit two months ago). His height is 38 inches (the same as his visit two months ago). His growth has not "fallen off the curve."

❓ What do you know so far? Well, Peter's vital signs are pretty normal except that his respiratory rate is a little fast. His weight is just below the 50th% for age, and his height is at the 50%. This is all pretty reassuring (except for the respiratory rate).

Peter's skin is clear (except the skin below his nose is slightly reddened). His nailbeds and tongue are pink. He allows you to do the entire exam while he sits on the examining table. His eyes are clear. The nasal mucosa is reddened and slightly swollen. There are no retractions, and the PMI is in the normal location. Air entry is adequate. There are a lot of upper airway noises. You can't hear expiration too well.

❓ What maneuver would help you to hear end expiration better? Yes. Gently squeeze Peter's chest. When you do this, you hear some faint, scattered wheezes at the bases.

There are no crackles or areas of decreased breath sounds. The cardiac and abdominal exams are within normal limits.

Peter points to his left ear for you to examine first. This ear has normal color, landmarks, and movement. So does the right one. (Ah, the serous otitis is resolved). While you look in his ears, you casually mention that Peter missed his "ear check." Mrs. Erlin looks surprised. Then she says, "Oh God, I forgot all about it." You reassure her that Peter's ears look fine now. When you examine his mouth and throat, Peter is able to "pant" for you, to visualize his pharynx. You note that there is clear mucus in the nasopharynx. The tonsils are 3 + in size. (Mrs. Erlin asks, "Why are his tonsils so big? Does that mean he'll need to have them removed?") They do not look inflamed. The rest of his mouth and pharynx are normal.

His neck is supple. There are some shotty anterior cervical lymph nodes. There are no abnormal nodes found anywhere else on his body. His musculoskeletal and gross neurologic exams are normal.

❓ What information does Peter's exam add? He does indeed have an upper respiratory infection (a "cold"), but he has a complication: some mild wheezing. He's breathing slightly faster than expected but doesn't seem to be in any respiratory distress. Now, I'll help you a little. The cough is most likely from both the postnasal drip and from the bronchospasm. Mild bronchospasm is not an uncommon complication of some viral respiratory infections. If this is Peter's first episode of wheezing (and it seems to be), he may not necessarily wheeze in the future. The tonsil size is not unexpected for a toddler with multiple upper respiratory infections. The size isn't worrisome as long as it doesn't interfere with swallowing or breathing (it doesn't). He doesn't have chronic ear disease.

You explain to Mrs. Erlin that Peter has a cold with some mild wheezing. For the stuffy nose, Peter may take a decongestant (he doesn't have to), and for the wheezing, he can take a bronchodilator. These should help his breathing and diminish his cough. You reaffirm that Peter's ears are normal now. Mrs. Erlin looks slightly better, but then she asks, "Does this mean he has asthma? Is that why he gets so many colds?"

You're getting in over your head. You respond, "I don't think so, but let me get my supervisor in to talk about that some more."

You've done really well so far, but you need some more help. You retreat to find your attending, to whom you report the results of the encounter so far. Dr. Grant, who knows the Erlins well, accompanies you back into the room. After greeting them, and commiserating about Peter's latest illness, she listens to Peter's chest and looks in his ears. She confirms your findings. She restates Mrs. Erlin's concerns about "asthma" but explains that some "very healthy" children wheeze once or twice with "colds." She adds,

"These children may not ever wheeze again. Sometimes they do, however, but since this is Peter's first experience it is really too early to tell. More importantly, let's look at how he's breathing today. He's really not having too difficult a time of it. His stuffy nose is giving him most of the trouble. And I'm happy that his ear is all better. Let's deal with how he looks right now. Let's also discuss your concern about why he's sick all the time."

Does Peter have any history or physical exam evidence for an ominous underlying cause for his "colds" (assuming he doesn't have asthma)? This is not a trick question. The answer is no. In fact his history and physical exam are very reassuring: His growth and development are absolutely normal! (extremely important information). He has had no unusual or serious infections. Five to six upper respiratory infections per year is "average" for many normal children. Parents are **extremely** relieved to hear this statistic. Children who are exposed to their first "group" situations will get more colds for a while until they "build up their immunity." Children in group day care seem to get more colds than those who are not in groups. Peter has experienced the same reaction to introduction to day care (and a new group of children) that many children experience.

His physical exam is reassuring too. There are no "unexpected" surprises. (Earlier in the text we mentioned that unexpected findings on physical exams, without historical information to clue us in first, are very rare!). Peter's otitis media is resolved. His tonsil size is compatible with his age and history. It is not evidence of a "bad" or "chronic disease" (his other lymphoid tissue is unremarkable). The wheezing is new. He may or may not ever wheeze again.

Mrs. Erlin actually smiles. She's feels a little better. Dr. Grant obtains some further "social history." Even though the Erlins have been undergoing a great deal of stress, Mrs. Erlin seems to have coped adequately up until now. This illness of Peter's constituted just one stress too many. Dr. Grant goes on to discuss the natural feelings of guilt, anger, and worry experienced by a concerned parent under circumstances like those experienced by the Erlin's. She points out how well Peter really seems to be doing. Finally, Dr. Grant offers future availability for Mrs. Erlin, to "come in and talk" if she feels she would like to do this. Mrs. Erlin responds gratefully that she will see how things are going.

Most of the information that you needed to

sort out the multiple problems of this clinical encounter were obtained by thorough history taking (including looking for hidden agendas) and good physical examination (including "plotting measurements"). As you gain more experience in pediatrics, you will increasingly realize the importance of these fundamental skills.

References

1. Solomon R. Pediatric experiences in year II clinical sciences. E. Lansing, Michigan: Department of Pediatrics and Human Development, College of Human Medicine, Michigan State University, 1986.
2. Brazelton TB. A child-oriented approach to toilet-training. Pediatrics 1962;29:121–128.
3. Galazka SS. Clinical magic and the art of examining children. Fam Pract 1984;18:229–232.
4. Moss JR. Helping young children cope with the physical examination. Pediatr Nurs 1981;March/April:17–20.
5. National Institutes of Health Consensus Development Conference Statement. Neurofibromatosis. U.S. Department of Health and Human Services Publications 1987;6:1–7.
6. Tunnessen WW. Cutaneous infections. Pediatr Clin North Am 1983;30:515–518.
7. American Academy of Pediatrics Committee on Practice and Ambulatory Medicine. Vision screening and eye examination in children. Pediatrics 1986;77:918–919.
8. Dworkin PH. The preschool child: developmental themes and clinical issues. Curr Probl Pediatr 1988;117–119.
9. Staheli LT. Torsional deformity. Pediatr Clin North Am 1977;24:802.
10. Staheli LT. Torsional deformity. Pediatr Clin North Am 1977;24:803–806.
11. Renshaw TS. Pediatric orthopedics. Philadelphia: W.B. Saunders Co., 1986.

CHAPTER **5**

School-Age

THE SCHOOL-AGE HISTORY
Student Task

1. Obtain a school-age history.

Most school-age children are old hands at clinical encounters. Your interaction is likely to go a lot smoother than with younger children. The five- to ten-year-old generally understands the purpose of the visit or hospitalization. She is also likely to be familiar with your instruments and the physical exam.

But, (there's always a but, isn't there?) bear in mind that she's coming to you with vivid memories of previous medical visits (remember this may be a plus or a minus). Second, her temperament is well established and visible. It will be easy to make friends if she is an outgoing and friendly child. If, on the other hand she is "shy" or "slow to warm up," securing her willing cooperation will be more challenging. Finally, remember that she may have a developmentally appropriate fear or reluctance.

Therefore, it will still pay to: **Prepare, Observe, and Modify.**

Emily Anne arrives for her "pre-kindergarten" health maintenance visit. You notice her in the hallway while Ellen screens her vision. Say, "hi" and tell her that you are going to do her check-up (most people still call it that). A review of her old chart reveals that she's had numerous episodes of otitis media. She has a mild case of eczema that's easy to control. Her brother, Charlie, is ten years old. During the past year (at problem visits) there have been several discussions, initiated by her mom, about intense sibling rivalry.

You review the **"five"** year flow sheet and note the **"ease of separation," "school readiness"** (including both the child's and parent's expectations) and **"peer interaction"** are appropriate topics for discussion. You also note that it's time for immunizations. **Preparation** has given you some important topics for discussion with mom. It has also provided you with topics easily discussed with this pre-kindergartener. While you are making friends, don't forget to **observe** her ease of separation, gender identity, and temperament or style. While you converse, listen to her speech for clarity and content. If she's extroverted and prepared, she may ask, "Am I going to get a shot today?" The four- to six-year-old has some real concerns about bodily harm. Answer truthfully, but soften your answer by telling her, "It won't happen until we're all finished; and I won't surprise you with it; afterwards, you'll get a reward for bravery."

If Emily's brother, Charlie is with her, pay attention to him, too. The five- or six-year-old may not object to her older brother's presence during the visit. However, if you're forewarned about intense sibling rivalry, it might be better to have him wait in the waiting room. This will make Emily's visit "special." On the other hand, some children at this age feel more at ease when an older sib remains. If your patient is eight or ten, it is appropriate to ask her if she would like some privacy. Some eight- or ten-year-olds will answer in the affirmative. When you increasingly involve your patient in direct conversation and allow her more choices during the encounter, you find out more about your patient. You compliment her and make her feel more grown up, and you begin to move the child into the ideal adult model of independent participation in the health care system.

Regardless of your patient's age, after a general opening question, begin your specific questions with familiar and comfortable subjects. For example, "What's good and bad about school?; Who is your most favorite teacher and why?; Who is your least favorite teacher and why?; What are your friends' names?; What do you like to do with your friends?; What do you do after school and on weekends;" Do you have any jobs around the house?; What are the rules at home?" Once you have achieved some rapport, you may proceed with more difficult questions such as, "What sorts of things make you happy? sad? worried?" For older children, you may continue with, "Some kids your age have tried drinking alcohol, or drugs; some have tried smoking; have your friends done this? have you? how do you feel about drinking alcohol? smoking? drugs?; have you noticed any changes in your body lately? **Modify** your questions as you proceed. Use the flow sheets and explanatory notes to remind you of topics. As children approach adolescence, you will want to focus more and more on the subjects of substance abuse and sexuality. By "paving the way" during middle childhood visits, with a nonjudgmental and matter-of-fact approach, you teach your patient that these are appropriate topics for discussion during visits with the doctor. In the explanatory notes, we will touch upon these topics briefly. More extensive discussion will be found in the next chapter.

Don't forget to include specific questions pertinent to the child's past medical history. For instance, ask Emily how her ears have been lately. She may not be able to answer this, but it will make her a participant in the discussion about medical problems as well as more routine subjects. This is an opportunity to educate as well as to question. You may clarify misconceptions or uncover hidden fears. This is also the time to ask her if she has any other somatic complaints, as these become increasingly common during middle childhood.

Early School Years Explanatory Notes: (Five Years through Six Years)

GENERAL CARE

Diet

What does the child eat during the course of a day? What does a typical breakfast consist of? What do snacks consist of? Are there any limits placed on food? Are there concerns about weight?

Sleep

How many hours a night does the child sleep? What is his bedtime? Are there "battles" over going to sleep? If so, how are these handled? Are there nighttime difficulties? (e.g., nightmares, night terrors, somnambulism).

Elimination

Has independence in bowel and bladder functioning been achieved? Are there problems (e.g., enuresis, encopresis, constipation or diarrhea)?

Safety

Does the child use a seat belt all the time? Has the child been instructed in fire safety and bicycle safety. Does he know how to swim? Is water play supervised at all times? If there is participation in an organized program is this program "approved" and well supervised? Is appropriate protective gear mandatory in this type of program (e.g., helmets for T-ball, or shin guards for soccer)? Does the child know what to do if approached by a stranger?

Play

What kind of play does the child enjoy most? Does this involve other children? Does he get regular physical exercise? Does he enjoy it? Does he have any hobbies (e.g., collec-

Table 5.1
History Flow Sheets: School Age

| Early School Age | History | | | Interval Updates | |
	General Care	Growth and Development	Developmental Milestones	General Health (ROS and PMH)	Family and Psycho-Social

Five Years	Diet habits
	Sleep
	  nighttime
	  problems
	Elimination
	  problems
	Safety
	  seatbelt/fire
	  bicycle/water
	  strangers
	Play
	  preferences
	T.V.
	Dental
		Affective
		Temperament
		Autonomy/
		Independence
		  ease of
		  separation
		Peer Interaction
		  relationships
		
		Gender Identity
		  fixed
		
		Cognitive
		  school readiness:
		  parent's
		    expectation,
		    child's reactions
		    school progress
		
		Physical
		  physician-child
		  relationship
			Tiptoes
			
			Dressing/
			  undressing
			  without
			  supervision
			
			Tell a simple
			  story
			
			Define at least
			  one word
			  (e.g., "ball,"
			  shoe)
			
			Beginning
			  understanding
			  of right/
			  wrong; rules
			
			Cuts and pastes
				Health Update
				
				Immunization
				  reactions
				  contraindications
				
				Somatic
				  complaints
				  (e.g., limb
				  pains)
				
				Habits
				
				Vision/Hearing
				
				Speech
					Family
					Status

Six Years	Diet habits
	Sleep problems
	Elimination
	  problems
	Safety
	  seatbelt/
	  bicycle
	  water/sports
	Play
	  preferences/
	  hobbies
	T.V.
	Dental
		Affective
		Temperament
		Autonomy/
		Independence
		  challenge of limits
		Peer interaction
		  relationships
		  peer influence
		
		Cognitive
		  school child/
		  parent reports
		
		Physical
		  physician/child
		  interaction
		  awareness of
		  body
			Skip
			
			Tie shoe laces
			
			Digit Span
			6-3-9-5
			7-5-1-4
			
			Copy
				Health Update
				Immunization
				  reactions
				  contraindications
				Somatic
				  complaints
				Habits
				Vision/Hearing
				Speech
					Family
					Status

tions)? How much television does he watch? Are there any limitations imposed on time or content of television viewing?

Dental Care

Does the child brush his or her teeth and have regular dental checkups?

GROWTH AND DEVELOPMENT

Affective Development

Temperament. What type of a child is he (e.g., outgoing, shy, fearful, "slow to warm up," etc.)? Is he "easy" or "difficult?" How do parents respond to difficulties?

Table 5.1—*continued*

Preadoles-cent	History			Interval Updates	
	General Care	Growth and Development	Developmental Milestones	General Health (ROS and PMH)	Family and Psycho-Social

Eight Years	Diet habits
	Sleep habits
	Elimination
	  problems
	Exercise habits
	Safety habits/
	  risk taking
	Hobbies
	  preferences
	Dental
		Affective
		Temperament
		Autonomy/
		  Independence
		  declaration of
		  independence
		Peer Interaction
		  ↑ peer
		  influence
		  segregation
		  with same sex/
		  "best friend"
		  confront w/
		  authority
		
		Cognitive
		school progress:
		  child/parent
		  reports
		  concrete
		  operations
		
		Physical
		  prepubertal:
		  changes?
		  physician/child
		  interaction
		  sex education
			Hop twice on
			  each foot
			
			Finger
			  opposition
			  (5 seconds)
			
			Digit span
			  5-3-8-1-6
			  6-4-3-9-1
			
			Copy
				Health Update
				Immunization
				  reactions
				  contraindications
				Somatic
				  complaints
				Puberty
				Habits
				Vision/Hearing
				Speech
					Family
					Status

Ten Years	Health Habits
	Diet
	Sleep
	Exercise
	Safety
	  risk taking
	  substance
	  abuse
	
	Dental
	Hobbies
		Affective
		Temperament
		Autonomy/
		  Independence
		  increasing
		  responsibility
		Peer interaction
		  peer influence
		Cognitive
		school progress
		
		Physical
		  sex education
		  pre-puberty →
		  early puberty
			Heel-Toe
			  eyes closed
			
			Make a ball
			
			Copy
				Health Update
				Immunizations
				  reactions
				  contraindications
				Somatic
				  complaints
				Puberty
				Habits
				Vision/Hearing
				Speech
					Family
					Status

Autonomy/Independence. Are there still some difficulties with separation? When do these occur? How are these handled? What kinds of limits are imposed? Are "limits" challenged or tested frequently? How does he "act out" (e.g., talk "fresh," disobey, aggressive, etc.)? How is this handled?

Peer Interaction. How does the child get along with other children? How much time does he spend playing with other children outside of school? Does he have a best friend? If there are difficulties, how are these handled?

Gender Identity.   Is gender identity fixed? ("Are you a boy or a girl?")

Cognitive Development

If the child has not yet begun school, explore both parental and child reactions to approaching school entry. What are the parent's perceptions of the child's readiness for school?

If the child has begun formal schooling, explore both parental and child reactions to school. Ask the child if he enjoys school. Ask him what he likes best about school and what he dislikes about school. Ask the parent how their child is doing in school. Inquire about areas of strength and difficulty. If there are areas of difficulty, how have these been addressed by both the school and the parents? How does the child feel about these difficulties? How many days was the child absent so far this year? What was the explanation for the absences?

School now becomes the most important parameter for a child's cognitive functioning. Monitoring of affective and physical development will also increasingly be linked with school performance and participation. For instance: ease of separation will influence a child's initial adjustment to school. Second, the child's temperamental style will influence initial school adjustment. The "slow to warm up" child will need special attention and extra "time" at the start of school.[1]

Physical Development

As we have previously discussed, the nature of the child-physician relationship begins to change at this age. Along with increased understanding of the encounter by the patient, you may see some "silliness" or "fear" at certain junctures. These may be related to an increased awareness of his or her own body. Deal with these in an understanding, but "matter of fact" manner. Respect modesty, even at this age.

DEVELOPMENTAL MILESTONES

Can the five-year-old walk on tip toes? Does he dress and undress himself without supervision (except tying shoes)? Can he tell a simple story? or define a simple word (e.g., ball, shoe, etc.)? Is he beginning to understand right and wrong? Does he "cut and paste"?[2]

Can the six-year-old skip? Does he know how to tie his shoe laces? Can he repeat 4 numbers in sequence back to the examiner after hearing them once? Can he copy an age appropriate figure? (see flow sheet)

GENERAL HEALTH

Obtain an interval update.

Immunizations

At the pre-kindergarten visit, there may be booster immunizations scheduled (i.e., DTP, OPV). Review previous reactions and contraindications.

Somatic Complaints

Are there "limb" pains or other frequent somatic complaints? How are these handled?

Habits

Does the child have any particular habits (e.g., nailbiting, thumbsucking, tics, etc.). When does the child engage in this habit? How does the child (and parents) view the habit? Has any attempt been made to extinguish it? What method was tried and what was the result?

Vision/Hearing

Do the parents think that their child sees and hears normally? If the child has been "screened" elsewhere, what were the results of this screening?

Speech

Is the child's speech clear? Are there dysfluencies? (Ask for specific examples). What percentage of the child's speech is difficult to understand or involves the dysfluency? How have these been handled?

FAMILY/PSYCHO-SOCIAL

Obtain an interval update. When the child enters the school system, there are often dramatic changes in the household. For instance, mother may return to work outside of the home. This may mean new childcare arrangements. The five- or six-year-old may not only have to adjust to school, but may also have to adjust to a new babysitter. Any problems? How is everyone doing? Is there special "quiet" time at the end of the day, set aside for parents and children to talk? Review parent-parent, parent-child, and sibling relationships.

Include family interactions in your **observations.** Listen not only to what is said, but how it is said. Does the parent encourage, compliment, and support her child? Or, is she overly critical, demanding, or rigid? Does the parent seem happy? sad? Is limit setting present? Is it appropriate? How does she handle issues between siblings?

Pre-Adolescent Years Explanatory Notes: (Eight Years through Ten Years)

During this age period, children begin to have increased self-reliance for personal needs. Most are capable of handling increased personal freedoms, choices, and obligations. However, this independence should be accompanied by a clear set of rules and obligations. The manner of "personal habits" that are learned during this period, is likely to strongly impact on future adult lifestyles.

GENERAL CARE

Diet

What does the child eat during the course of the day? What does a typical breakfast consist of? What do snacks consist of? Are there any limits placed on food? Does the child (or parents) actively try to control his or her weight? If so, by what methods?

Sleep

What are the child's sleep habits? What is his or her bedtime? Is sleep time adequate? Are there nighttime difficulties (e.g., nightmares, night terrors, somnambulism)?

Elimination

Are bowel and bladder habits regular and predictable? Are there any problems (e.g., enuresis, encopresis, constipation)?

Exercise

Does the child get regular physical exercise? How is this accomplished? Does he or she enjoy physical exercise? Does he do well in sports? Which ones in particular?

Safety

Does the child use a seat belt at all times? Does the child behave in a responsible and safe fashion? Does he take risks with his body that frighten or concern parents (e.g., fire setting, refusing to use protective equipment during athletics, swimming without an adult present, etc.)? Has there been discussion about and/or involvement in: drugs, alcohol, or smoking? Do parents limit access to dangerous machinery? If there is participation in an organized athletic program, is this program "approved" and well-supervised? Is appropriate protective gear mandatory in this type of program?

Dental

Does he brush his or her teeth and have regular dental checkups? Does he get a lot of cavities?

Hobbies

What does the child enjoy doing in his free time? Does he have hobbies? Does he read for pleasure?

GROWTH AND DEVELOPMENT
Affective Development

Temperament. What is the child like? Does he seem happy? Is he outgoing or withdrawn? Is he moody or unpredictable? Is he worried about anything? What is he afraid of?

Autonomy/Independence. Is the child becoming visibly more independent of parents and more involved in peer values and interests? Are there major conflicts between child and parents? How are these handled? What is communication like between child and parents? Does the child have increasing responsibilities at home (e.g., chores)?

Peer Interaction. What are the child's friends like? What common interests do they share? How much time does he spend with them? Does he play with children of the opposite sex? Does he have a best friend? Are there major conflicts with figures of authority besides parents (e.g., teachers, etc.)? Have there been problems with fighting, stealing, lying, etc.?

Cognitive Development

How is school going? (Ask both child and parents). What grades does he or she get? Has he or she had to repeat a grade? Why? What does he like best about school? What does he dislike the most about school? If there are areas of difficulty, how have these problems been addressed? How many days of school has he or she missed thus far this year? What were the reasons for the absences? "Is the child able to focus on multiple aspects of a problem, establish hierarchies and use logic? Is he or she able to "see" the viewpoints of others? (concrete operations)"[3]

Physical Development

Have issues of sexual development and sexuality been discussed between parents and child? What are parent's plan for handling these issues? How aware is child about these issues (particularly of upcoming changes to his or her own body)? Do parents or child have any questions or concerns about these issues?

For the older child, has he or she noticed any changes in his/her body yet (e.g., breast buds, body hair, or growth spurt)? Does she understand what is happening to her and what will happen in the future?

Does the child wish to be examined alone today? Is the child aware that in the future the majority of the visit will be spent without parent present?

DEVELOPMENTAL MILESTONES
(see flow sheet)

Can the eight-year-old hop on each foot twice, while smoothly alternating one foot to the other? Can he oppose thumb and fifth finger, then each other successive finger with thumb in rapid sequence (within five seconds)? Can he accurately repeat five digits? Can he copy an age-appropriate figure?

Can the ten-year-old stand heel to toe in a straight line with his eyes closed for fifteen seconds? Can he crumple up paper into a ball (without using a table surface) in 5 seconds using the dominant hand? (and 7 seconds using the nondominant hand?). Can he copy an age-appropriate figure?

GENERAL HEALTH

Obtain an interval update.

Immunization

If immunizations are scheduled, review patient and household contraindications. This includes reviewing reactions to prior immunizations.

Somatic Complaints

Does the child have any chronic complaints? If so, how have these been handled? Does the problem interfere with sleep or activity?

Pubertal Changes
(see Physical Development)

You may choose to discuss signs of puberty when you discuss general health (as part of your review of systems); or you may have already included this subject as part of a discussion on development in general.

Habits

Does the child have any particular habits? (e.g., nailbiting, thumbsucking, compulsions, etc.). If so, how does the child (and parents) view the habits? Do friends tease him about it? Have any attempts been made to extinguish the behavior? What method was tried and what was the result?

Vision/Hearing

Does the child see and hear normally? If the child has been "screened" elsewhere, what were the results of this screening?

Speech

Is the child's speech clear? Are there dysfluencies? If there are speech problems, how have these been handled?

FAMILY/PSYCHO-SOCIAL

Obtain an interval update. Any problems? How is everyone doing? Review parent-child and sibling relationships if these have not been explored previously.

THE PHYSICAL EXAM OF THE SCHOOL-AGE CHILD

Student Task

1. Examine a school-age child.

As we've already discussed, most school-age children are cooperative. As long as you keep up a running conversation with them about subjects with which they are familiar and interested, you've got it made.

The "helter skelter" order isn't usually necessary. The willing child can be examined in a "head to toe" fashion, similar to adults. The important differences in expected findings and in areas of concentration will be discussed as we go along.

Some five- and six-year-olds won't mind being examined in their underwear and some will. The older child may be modest.

Offer her a gown to go over her underpants, and expose only one area at a time. A drape is helpful too (e.g., when you examine her abdomen: pull the gown up to expose the abdomen, after covering the bottom half of her body with a drape). Taking the extra time to address this modesty sends an important message to your young patient: that you take her seriously. She, in turn, will take you more seriously, too.

Attention to modesty will also enhance your patient's feeling of being in control. This may be amplified by giving her choices as you proceed and by alerting her to what comes next. Earlier, we discussed the issue of having siblings present during the exam. The nine- or ten-year-old in particular will appreciate being able to make this choice. Allow other choices as you go along, such as "Now I'm going to check your ears. Which ear should I look in first?"; "Now I'm going to examine your throat. See if you can open your mouth really wide so I don't need to use a tongue blade," etc.

Even though the **encounter in this age group usually goes smoothly, there may be some exceptions.** These will be:[15]

1. The younger child who is still experiencing **difficulties with separation,**
2. The extremely **shy** (or "slow to warm up child"),
3. The child who has had many **painful or scary previous medical experiences,**
4. The child who has been **physically or sexually abused,**
5. The **"out of control"** child who doesn't respond to normal limit setting,
6. The child who is **very ill.**

You may or may not be forewarned about some of these problems in the history. If you've done a reasonably thorough job at history taking, you may have had a suspicion before the physical began. Sometimes, not until you've begun the exam do you encounter an "unexpectedly" uncooperative patient. If this happens, take a deep breath and try to analyze the situation.[15] This is why **preparation, observation, and modification** apply to **all** age groups! We've already discussed how to handle the child with separation anxiety. The "slow to warm up" child and the child who is afraid because of previous experience can be dealt with in a similar fashion to younger children. Proceeding slowly and cautiously, using reassurance and explanations, usually works for these children. The advantage you have over younger children is their increased level of cognition. The seven- or eight-year-old can usually understand logical statements and reason.

If you find you cannot gain cooperation, even after the above approach, you should ask yourself, "Why not?" You might be dealing with a child who has difficulty with all types of limit setting ("out of control"). Some of these children have not had reasonable limit setting at home. There will likely be some clues to this earlier in your encounter. As you obtained the history, you may have **observed** interaction which suggested this problem. The parent may complain that there is a great deal of acting out behavior or "he doesn't ever listen to me." Previous issues of "limit setting" may be documented in the chart. If you suspect this is the case (after eliminating some of the other causes listed), try some limit setting of your own. You may need to ask the parent to leave the room. Tell your patients that after the exam is completed, you will allow the parent to come back into the room. This is usually a difficult judgment to make, especially at an early stage of training. If you need assistance (after you've thought this through), don't be reluctant to discuss this with your supervisor.

The child who has been physically or sexually abused may be uncooperative for the general physical exam, or just during the genital exam. If the abuse is known, and the purpose of the visit is to document the presence of physical stigmata of abuse, then you will need to seek assistance from your supervisor. Sometimes the patient hasn't told anyone yet. How do you distinguish between the normal child who naturally resists having her genitals examined and the

child who has been abused? It's not necessarily easy. Often, in the case of abuse, **something** in the history **doesn't fit,** either because there are behavioral issues, compliance problems, etc. There may be a history of prior neglect or abuse. There may be a history of an older sibling having been abused. In the case of a nonabused child, you will usually achieve success if you back off for a moment, explain what you need to do, have mom close at hand and try again. If your suspicions are aroused, obtain some further history before proceeding.

You will not be seeing medically unstable patients by yourself. You might, however, be assigned to examine a very ill but "stable" child. Follow the guidelines presented in the introductory chapter, in the section on the "pediatric ward," adapting your exam to the developmental level and condition of your patient.

More commonly, you may encounter a very uncomfortable, but not critically ill, child. Examples of these types of patients are children with acute abdominal pain or children with streptococcal pharyngitis. Children in middle childhood are remarkably cooperative, even when they are in pain. But attention to modesty and explanations should not be overlooked. If you encounter obstructive behavior, be forgiving and forget the parts of the exam that aren't necessary. However, if something is crucial (like examining the posterior pharynx in a child with a stiff neck . . . remember the peritonsillar abscess that was missed?) . . . be firm, and ask for assistance if required.

Continue to **observe** parent-child interaction, both physical and verbal. Are there signs of a supportive relationship?; or is there "distance" or excessive criticism?

Measurements

Before you begin, plot height and weight on the growth charts. Middle childhood is a period of steady, relatively slow growth with an actual slowing in rate just before adolescence. The beginning of the period of rapid adolescent growth (the "growth spurt") begins as early as 9½ (range 9½ − 14½) in girls and 10½ (range 10½−16) in boys. (The growth spurt peaks at approximately age 12 in girls and 14 in boys.) During middle childhood, children tend to grow about 2 inches per year and 7 lbs. per year. You don't need to remember the numbers. Be extra vigilant in plotting the findings on the growth charts and being sure that weight gain continues to "follow the curve." This is a "high risk" period for the development of obesity (especially in inactive children). Obesity is defined in a variety of ways using either growth charts (e.g., plot weight vs. age or weight vs. height) or triceps skinfold thickness (as measured by calipers). Values greater than 2 standard deviations above the mean or values greater than the 95% using any of these references are generally defined as obesity. In an infant, visual assessment for obesity is sometimes inaccurate. By the time the child reaches school age, if you think a child "looks" obese, you are probably correct.

You will examine some children with excessively short (less than the fifth percentile) or excessively tall (greater than the ninety-fifth percentile) stature. There are a variety of etiologies for either finding, depending on growth **pattern,** family history and associated medical problems (e.g., endocrine abnormalities, dysmorphic features, systemic illness, etc.) You will learn more about these entities during your clinical rotations, but you have already acquired the skills to perform most of the workup for either tall or short stature, a careful history and physical exam.

Ask your patient to take a seat on the examining table. **Wash your hands.**

Skin

Observe color and turgor. Note and describe rashes and birthmarks. During your pediatric encounters, you will see many eruptions that are new to you. We don't have space to discuss them all. In addition, even classic rashes sometimes present atypically. So, how do you learn to identify what you are seeing?

The first step, always, is to describe in detail what the rash looks like. Describe the **location and distribution** of the rash. Find out when and where on the body it began and what the **pattern of spread** was. Then describe the **characteristics of individual lesions.** Statements to include are: **number** of lesions (e.g., few, many) . . . **types** of lesions (e.g., papules, macules, pustules, vesicles, ulcers) . . . **color** of lesions (e.g., red, honey colored, flesh colored) . . . **characteristics** of lesions (e.g., blanching, nonblanching) . . . **distribution** of lesions (e.g., scattered, clustered, contiguous) . . . **symptoms** (e.g., itchy, painful). When you can accurately describe an eruption and combine that data with history, you will narrow-down the diagnostic possibilities considerably. (It is also then possible to look up the answer in a book.)

Itchy rashes constitute a large proportion of pediatric dermatologic problems. You already know about several itchy rashes: eczema and varicella. Other itchy conditions that look the same in children as in adults are: hives, insect bites, and contact dermatitis. Another that is **very** common in children is the rash of **scabies** (Figure 5.1). Scabies lesions may be papular, pustular, or papulovesicular. The parent or child frequently reports intense itching, especially at night (this is an important clue). Family members may have the same symptoms. Clusters of lesions may be found anywhere on the body but concentrate on: the hands, particularly the flexoral aspects of the wrists, the folds of the body, particularly the groin, finger webs and axillae, and also on the feet and buttocks. There are numerous excoriations. If you are fortunate, you will spot a linear burrow made by the etiologic organism: the mite. The linear burrow is pretty much diagnostic of scabies (but it's not too common). A diagnosis of scabies can be confirmed microscopically by scraping typical lesions and then identifying mites, ova, or fecal material. Pediatricians usually make this diagnosis clinically, as the success rate of the microscopic exam (in our hands) is low.

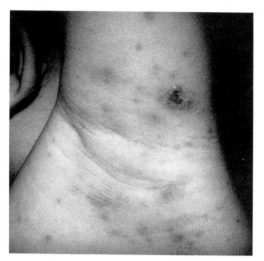

Figure 5.1. Scabies lesions in the axilla. Photo courtesy of Douglas H. MacGilpin, M.D.

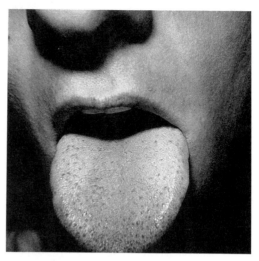

Figure 5.2. Strawberry tongue of scarlet fever. Photo courtesy of Stanley F. Glazer, M.D.

The other rash (that may be itchy) and is very common and important to recognize is the rash of **scarlet fever.** Group A beta hemolytic streptococcus is a significant pharyngeal pathogen in the school-age child. Some strep organisms elaborate a toxin which produces a rash that accompanies the pharyngitis. In these cases, the illness is called scarlet fever. The classic rash of scarlet fever consists of many tiny papules against a background of erythema. The rash most often begins on the face and neck and rapidly proceeds caudally to involve the trunk and extremities. The eruption feels a bit like "sandpaper." There is accentuation of the rash in the flexural creases (called **Pastia's** lines), and there is circumoral (around the lips) pallor. The rash on the tongue coats it white (white strawberry tongue). It then becomes denuded and thus, appears to have tiny red papules; this is called a **red strawberry** tongue (Figure 5.2). Days to weeks after the infection, the hands and feet may peel and the rest of the body may have a fine scale.

Another skin finding that is very common, is **bruising.** Active toddlers and school-age children frequently have multiple purpuric lesions on the anterior surfaces of the lower extremities. The bruises come in varying shades of purple to yellow, correlating with the time of previous injury. Let's face it, kids are very active and pretty careless. They collide with objects and people frequently. Parents, aware that "easy bruisability" might have some ominous etiologies (e.g., leukemia or bleeding dyscrasia) frequently point these bruises out and ask for reassurance. If the patient is active and healthy, has a normal physical exam, and has no history or family history reflecting a problem with bleeding or bruising, and has minimal bruising in other areas of the body, you will be able to reassure the parent. If there are a lot of other bruises, or something in the history or physical exam isn't right (e.g., a history of increasing fatigue, weight loss . . . or an enlarged spleen), there may be something else going on. When a **bruise has an unusual appearance** (e.g., linear, looped, or small and round), an **implausible location** (e.g., on the back, scalp or in a stocking-glove distribution), or when the **history either doesn't fit the injury** (e.g., a child with a black eye whose parent tells you "he fell down the stairs") **or the development ability of the child,** the question of **intentional injury** should be raised. If there is a history of **prior injury** or there has been an **unexplained delay in seeking medical**

care for a significant injury, such bruises further raise the question of intentional injury. My rule of thumb when I encounter such a situation during a physical exam is to casually ask the patient (if he is old enough to answer) or the parent, "How did that bruise happen?" **Observe** him (and his parent) while you listen to the answer.

Head/Hair

Assess the head for general appearance. Feel for prominences. Inspect the hair, including eyebrows, and look carefully at the scalp. **Alopecia** (lack of hair in areas where it is normally present) has many causes in childhood. In middle childhood, **traction alopecia** is a common cause. This is secondary to prolonged traction from pony tail holders or tight braiding. While this may seem obvious to you right now, it will not necessarily occur to you in the office if the child's hair isn't in the offending holder when you are performing the exam. If you see localized alopecia, especially in a female, ask about this particular etiology. Other common causes of localized alopecia are: fungal infections (**tinea capitis**) (Figure 5.3) and **alopecia areata**

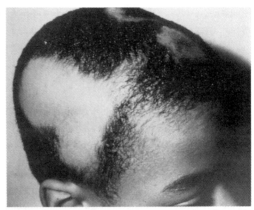

Figure 5.4. Alopecia areata. Reproduced with permission. Fleisher GR, Ludwig S., eds. Textbook of pediatric emergency medicine. 2nd. ed. Baltimore: Williams & Wilkins, 1988:801.

(Figure 5.4) (this may or may not be associated with thyroid or autoimmune disease). Alopecia areata presents as a circumscribed path completely devoid of hair, whose skin surface is smooth and devoid of stubble (in contrast to tinea capitis). Exclamation point hairs which are short and stubby, may be found at the edge of the bald patch. Sometimes there is a more diffuse thinning rather than a localized patch of alopecia. This may be associated with a systemic illness or may, like localized alopecia, be idiopathic. When you encounter alopecia, scrape the edge of a patch and pluck several hairs out. Examine the scrapings and hair roots with KOH preparation under the microscope for fungus. Fungal infections on the head require microbiologic confirmation, especially if systemic antifungal treatment is considered. Before we leave the hair, we ought to mention the school-age child's parent's nightmare: head lice. Head lice is an extremely common problem in school-age children, encouraged by the close physical contact and "sharing" of hats in this age group. Most children with head lice are diagnosed over the phone and don't make it to the doctor's office. Nevertheless, you will see it occasionally. The nits (or eggs) hand on tightly to the hair shaft and look like tiny white particles which don't pull off (like dandruff will). The scalp is pruritic.

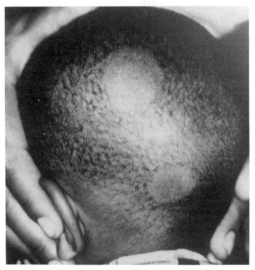

Figure 5.3. Tinea capitis. Reproduced with permission. Fleisher GR, Ludwig S., eds. Textbook of pediatric emergency medicine. 2nd. ed. Baltimore: Williams & Wilkins, 1988:798.

Face

Remember to begin with a general overall impression before zeroing in. Is the child alert and oriented? happy, anxious, sad? Is there something unusual about his appearance?

The "classic" **facies** of a child with **upper respiratory tract allergy** is so characteristic that pediatricians can make this diagnosis from the doorway. See if you can, too. (Figure 5.5) This child has a **long face** with **shadows under the eyes** (from venous engorgement), horizontal skin creases under the lower lids (called **Dennie's lines**), a horizontal crease just above the tip of his nose (called a **nasal pleat**) (from wiping his drippy nose in an upward fashion) and an **open mouth** (because nasal congestion makes it difficult to breath through his nose). The shadows under his eyes are called: **allergic shiners,** and the characteristic upward nose wipe with the palm of the hand is called the **allergic salute.** Although the terms are somewhat comical, the condition is not. These children are plagued with a "constant cold" and benefit from aggressive treatment for their symptoms. A similar constellation of facial findings is also seen in children with chronic adenoid enlargement and obstruction.

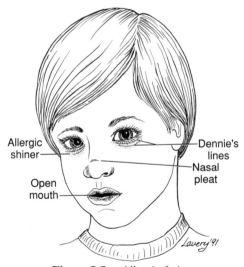

Figure 5.5. Allergic facies.

Eyes

Assess shape, size, and symmetry. Continue as previously discussed, by concentrating on individual structures one at a time. Note pupillary reaction to light and accommodation. Ask about visual difficulties in addition to screening for acuity. Children 5 years of age or older should read a majority of the 20/30 line. Failure to do that, or a two-line difference between eyes (even in the normal range) warrants referral.[4] If vision screens are performed at each well child visit and have been normal, and the history doesn't suggest a problem, then you may skip objective testing in the 10-year-old.[5] Color vision should be assessed at least one time during the school-age years. The recommended equipment utilizes special pseudo-isochromatic plates.

Sadly, an occasional muscle imbalance goes undetected until the kindergarten age group. (the likelihood of full sight correction at this late age is diminished). Assess the corneal light reflex and perform the alternate cover test. Assess the range of extra ocular motion.

Examine the fundus. Have the parent hold up an object or a hand for the child to focus on. Tell the child to try to "see through" your head and look toward the object. Tell him **not** to look at the light; that is, if the light gets in his way, he should continue to concentrate on looking towards the object. Darkened rooms facilitate fundoscopic exams. With practice, you can perform an adequate fundus exam even in a five-year-old. If the history suggests a visual or cranial nerve problem, perform a visual field exam by confrontation.

❓ **You suspect your patient has suffered a basilar skull fracture. He has a Battle's sign. What's that? Ecchymosis behind the ear. He also has blood behind the tympanic membrane which is also a sign of basilar skull fracture. He also has a third finding associated with this problem, a *Racoon's sign*. These are ecchymoses around the eyes.**

Ears

Inspect the external ear and feel behind the ear. Inquire about complaints related to the ears and hearing. Check to see that the hearing screen is normal. If a normal hearing screen is obtained at age 5, and the history does not suggest a problem, you may defer objective screening at ages 6–10.[5] Pull back on the auricle.

❓ If your patient complains of pain when you pull back on the auricle, and the ear is draining fluid, what's wrong? Very likely, the child has "swimmer's ear" or otitis externa. Otitis media (without drum rupture) doesn't produce these findings.

In this age group, you can continue with otoscopy at this time. Pull the pinna up and back. Examine the canal as you gently advance the otoscope. Examine the drum for color, translucency, and landmarks. Insufflate and observe the movement of the drum. The correct ear speculum size for school age children is usually a "4."

As we've mentioned previously, otitis externa is uncommon in young children, probably because of their infrequent head submersion during swimming. In the school-age group, however, otitis externa is a common summertime problem. With otitis externa, the canal is red, swollen, and exquisitely tender; there will purulent material in the canal. Chances are, you won't be able to advance your otoscope very far, because your patient won't let you. You can try, if you get cooperation. The chief reason to pursue this is to exclude the possibility that the drainage originates from an otitis media with drum rupture (the other is to exclude a foreign body irritation). Sometimes, there is so much drainage in the canal, that the drum cannot be adequately visualized. In this instance, the decision about treatment will be based on assessment of the total picture (e.g., presence of fever and other systemic signs would make you favor otitis media; or a history of swimming, pain on movement of the pinna, and no systemic signs, would make you favor otitis externa).

❓ The canal is "clear." You have visualized the ear drum, and it is pearly grey and semi-transparent. You insufflate. The drum doesn't move. You try again, It still doesn't move. Why not? First check to see that you have a good seal around the speculum. You do. Second, there could be fluid behind the drum (in an asymptomatic child this would most likely be "serous" fluid). You see no evidence of any fluid. Could there still be fluid? Yes. Drums that are thickened and scarred (usually from recurrent infection) also don't move very well in response to insufflation. But, this drum doesn't appear thickened or scarred. But wait, look again. You really haven't inspected the "whole" drum. When you do, you notice a *perforation in the eardrum*. A perforated drum is the other common reason (besides fluid behind the drum or scarring) for lack of movement upon insufflation. Perforations of the tympanic membrane are either spontaneous or induced (by trauma). Spontaneous perforations occur most often when a bulging, inflamed eardrum spontaneously "drains" when the pressure buildup exceeds a certain limit. These spontaneous perforations associated with otitis media usually occur in the central portion of the drum, although they may occur in other parts too. Induced perforations (besides those performed by otolaryngologists) most commonly occur when a child (or parent) sticks something smaller than an elbow into the ear canal and accidentally perforates the eardrum. This often happens when someone is trying to "clean" out the canal, with a Q-tip or bobby pin. The real danger of this is that not all areas of the drum heal spontaneously when perforated. Fortunately, spontaneous ruptures from otitis media usually do. Traumatic perforations are not that predictable. When the perforation isn't in the center of the drum, and/or associated with a middle ear infection, suspect an etiology other than infection.

The point of the above "exercise" was to teach you to look at the entire drum. If you don't really inspect the whole tympanic membrane, you may miss a perforation or even an air fluid level. The tympanic membrane perforation in the accompanying figure (see Figure 5.6) resulted from a chronic middle ear infection. One final point about ear drums. (Remember, I mentioned how much there is to learn about this commonly affected organ?). Eustachian tube swelling (called dysfunction), which occurs with the inflammation associated with upper respiratory infection or allergy, interferes with the normal pressure equalization in the middle ear. The result may be a **retracted drum** (the opposite

of a bulging drum) that will also not move very well upon insufflation (especially won't move "in" on squeezing the bulb). Practice looking for all of the findings we have discussed, and perform pneumatic otoscopy on all cooperative children, even if they are asymptomatic. You may find an abnormality. Second, you will do a much better job on the more challenging younger patient.

Nose

Check for patency and drainage. Examine the mucosa, turbinates, and septum. The lower turbinates may be swollen if chronically inflamed (e.g., from infection). These may be confused with nasal polyps, which are not common in childhood, and if present are found between the middle and lower turbinates. True nasal polyps may be a presenting sign of cystic fibrosis.

Mouth and Pharynx

Inspect the anterior surfaces of the mouth and inspect general oral hygiene. This is always the perfect opportunity to ask about the dentist (and review speech clarity and content in your mind.) Smell the breath (more about this shortly).

Primary teeth shedding begins at around age 6, usually with the lower central incisors. Eruption of permanent teeth begins at approximately the same age with replacements for the lower central incisors as well as eruptions of the first permanent molars behind the primary molars. Shedding and eruption of permanent replacements for the upper central and lower lateral incisors occurs a year later between ages 7 and 8. A year after that (8 to 9), the upper lateral incisors are shed and replaced. Following this feverish oral activity, there is a period of quiescence for several years, after which the cuspids and primary molars are shed. The first bicuspids erupt at about age 10. I included the details for you to get a sense of the expected pattern; memorization isn't necessary.

Inspect hygiene, spacing and **occlusion.** Ask the child to bite down. The top teeth should overlap the bottom teeth all the way

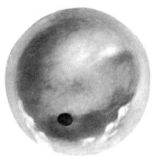

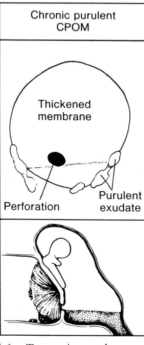

Figure 5.6. Tympanic membrane perforation associated with chronic otitis media. Reproduced with permission. Fleisher GR, Ludwig S., eds. Textbook of pediatric emergency medicine. 2nd. ed. Baltimore: Williams & Wilkins, 1988:428.

Chronic purulent
CPOM

Thickened
membrane

Perforation

Purulent
exudate

around. Make sure that the child is biting on the back teeth.

Inspect for oral ulcers. Many viral diseases are accompanied by multiple oral ulcers. What about the child who has only one or few oral ulcers? These are most likely aphthous ulcers or chancre sores. You will find these on fixed mucosa (e.g., palate or gingivae). These may be confused with the ulcers of recurrent herpes infection which are somewhat smaller and usually occur on moveable mucosa (e.g., on the vermillion border of the lip). Treatment of either is mostly supportive.

Ask your patient to open wide and inspect the tongue, palate, uvula, tonsils, and posterior pharynx. A child in this age group may be very cooperative for this exam. You may not need to use a tongue depressor in order to visualize the posterior structures. If you do use one, try placing it on the anterior two-thirds of the tongue, thus avoiding production of a gag response. (You really only need to place it more posteriorly when a child is totally uncooperative). Earlier, I mentioned that group A beta hemolytic strep is an important pathogen in this age group. The "classic" strep throat is heralded by bright red swollen tonsils and pharynx, with a yellowish tonsillar exudate, petechiae on the posterior palate, and foul smelling breath. This is accompanied by fever and swollen, tender anterior cervical lymph nodes.

❓ **What about the tongue? That's right. Some strep infections (scarlet fever) are accompanied by a "strawberry" tongue. When attempting to determine the etiology of pharyngitis, the problem you encounter is that infections caused by viruses may also be accompanied by bright red tonsils, exudate, and palatal petechiae.**

"Bad breath" not only accompanies pharyngitis and poor oral hygiene but is also a sign of sinusitis. If you see a slight amount of pharyngeal or tonsillar erythema and purulent postnasal drainage in a child with halitosis and fever (with or without a headache), think about the diagnosis of sinusitis.

❓ **What about the child who's feeling fine, has an otherwise normal examination, but has "kissing" tonsils? (4+ in size). We spoke about large tonsils during Peter's office visit. As long as there is no evidence of infection and breathing and swallowing are not affected, there is no need to worry. This is a common normal finding. When reassuring parents, check also to see that the tonsils look basically symmetric (a unilateral enlargement might signal an underlying infection or, rarely, a tumor). You will notice the variability in "peaking" of tonsillar size as you examine more and more children during middle childhood. If there has been chronic infection or overstimulation for any reason (e.g., allergy), tonsillar size may "peak" well before the average ages of 8 to 10.**

Neck

Inspect for bulges, head tilts and thyromegaly. After inspection, palpate the neck all around. Note shoddy nodes where present and all nodes that are enlarged beyond what you expect normally. Palpate the thyroid gland. This becomes slightly palpable (even when not enlarged) in the preadolescent. Palpate in the same manner that you have been taught in adults.

Group A beta hemolytic strep pharyngitis is accompanied by enlarged and tender anterior cervical lymph nodes. Pharyngitis of viral etiology may be accompanied by enlarged cervical nodes, too. Epstein Barr infection (mononucleosis) is classically accompanied by a predominance of enlarged posterior cervical nodes. This is sometimes clinically useful when distinguishing between "strep" and "mono." This difference is not absolute; there are always exceptions.

Evaluate range of motion. The complaint of **stiff neck** becomes increasingly common as a child grows older. By this, I mean a **wry neck or muscular torticollis,** rather than the stiff neck associated with meningitis. How do you tell the difference? You begin history taking with special attention to antecedent and associated symptoms. For example, you inquire about signs of systemic illness (e.g., fever and headache) if you suspect meningitis, and you investigate for trauma, abruptness of onset, and absence of systemic symptoms when you suspect a muscular torticollis. The child with wry neck from muscle spasm will generally demonstrate a lateral head tilt in the direction away from the muscle spasm. He will have difficulty straightening his head out and or rotating his head past the midline towards the side of the spasm. Unlike the child with a stiff neck from meningitis, he will be able to flex his neck so that his chin touches his chest. There are several difficulties with this simplistic explanation. First, the child with either pharyngitis or cervical adenitis (who may have fever, irritability, and headache) may develop a wry neck on the basis of local inflammation. Second, a child with a "simple" wry neck may have a rotary subluxation of the atlantoaxial joint or, rarely, a fracture, tumor, or arthritis of the cervical spine. I don't mention these to confuse you (really!). This is just to remind you that a **very** careful history, physical examination, including vital signs and neurologic examination is necessary, as always. Radiologic and laboratory investigation may also be required.

Thorax and Upper Extremities

You need to assess blood pressure, palpate pulses, examine the thorax, breasts, upper extremities, heart, and lungs. In the older school age female, you can't be quite as cavalier about the order of these as you might be in a younger child or in a male. One possible order for these is: 1. **Obtain blood pressure and palpate pulses. 2. Ask her to remove the shirt or gown. Inspect and palpate chest. Ask her to replace the gown. Complete the upper extremity exam. 3. Auscultate the heart and lungs while she is sitting up. (Either auscultate before she replaces the shirt or gown; or, alternatively, auscultate underneath the gown once she has replaced it. Either way, do not auscultate on top of any clothing.) 4. Ask her to lie down.**

Complete your auscultation. Perform a breast exam.

With this order, she need only lie down one time. However, if you hear a murmur while she's sitting, you may want to listen several times over, in both the upright and recumbent positions. The school-age patient is cooperative enough to comply easily with your requests. Just make sure you tell her what you're doing, without alarming her unduly (e.g., "I just need to concentrate a little more on this part of the examination.")

Let's back track in order to emphasize a few points:

Obtain blood pressure and palpate pulses.

❓ **Can you guess what is the most common explanation for an elevated blood pressure in a child? (Don't get too fancy with your answer.) The most common explanation for an elevated blood pressure in a child, is inappropriate cuff size selection (too small). Review the criteria for cuff size selection in the *measurements* section of the first chapter. The second most common explanation (for an elevated systolic pressure) is anxiety.**

If you obtain an elevated reading with a correctly sized cuff, wait until you have finished your exam and repeat the measurement. You may even need to ask your patient to lie down in a darkened room for fifteen or twenty minutes and obtain the measurement a third time. If the blood pressure in the upper extremities is still elevated, measure it in the lower extremities (think about a coarctation of the aorta). You will learn more about further evaluation of hypertension during your clinical experiences, but don't fall into the trap of measuring incorrectly.

Ask her to remove the shirt or gown. Inspect and palpate chest. Ask her to replace the gown. Complete the upper extremity exam.

An adequate chest exam can't be performed through clothing. The older child may require some privacy during this part of the exam (either by drawing a drape or asking accompanying sibs or others (e.g., fathers of females) to step outside. Inspect clavicles, breasts, thorax, sternum, and upper extremities, including hands and fingers. Warm your hands. Palpate the clavicles and axillae. Search for thoracic asymmetries. For example, a precordial bulge may signify an underlying enlarged heart, or a prominence of one side of the chest may develop secondary to a scoliosis.

During middle childhood, the trunk thins out. The thoracic cage elongates, and the abdomen appears more scaphoid (than in toddlers), in the erect position. As a result, a pectus excavatum (or carinatum) may appear more noticeable in this age group than in younger children.

Inspect the breasts of both sexes. In females, normal breast development begins as early as age 8 (or as late as 13). Initial development may be asymmetric. If a patient or her family hasn't been warned ahead of time, there may be a doctor's visit in middle childhood for a "painful breast lump." This is most often a unilateral, normal breast bud signifying the onset of puberty. The Tanner system of staging pubertal development in both sexes will be described in detail in the adolescent chapter. Briefly, it is a method to describe and monitor progression of secondary sexual changes during puberty. "Tanner 1" (breasts, pubic hair, or genitalia) always signifies a prepubertal appearance. For breast development, this equals flat breasts with elevation of the papillae only. Most females develop Tanner 2 breasts prior to acquiring pubic hair (although the reverse order may also be within normal limits): the papillae and areola become elevated as a small mound and the areola widens.[6] The average age of acquiring Tanner 2 breasts in the U.S. is 10½; this coincides with the onset of the growth spurt. You will palpate breast tissue when your patient is supine.

Ask her to replace the gown. Evaluate upper extremity bulk, tone, strength, and range of motion.

Cardiorespiratory

During middle childhood the PMI gradually changes location. It moves (from left of the midclavicular line) to the midclavicular line between ages 4 to 6 and to the right of the midclavicular line at approximately age seven. It also moves downward from the 4th interspace to the 5th interspace by the age of seven.[7] Palpate the precordium, the PMI, and feel for thrills, heaves, or lifts.

Auscultate the heart and lungs while she is sitting up. (Either auscultate before she replaces the shirt or gown, or, alternatively, auscultate underneath the gown once she has replaced it. Either way, do not auscultate on top of any clothing.)

Auscultate for rate and rhythm, then listen to each sound individually. A third heart sound may be heard in diastole at the apex in many healthy children, particularly during middle childhood.[8] Without an associated pathologic murmur (e.g., the holosystolic murmur of mitral insufficiency), it is of no significance. A fourth heart sound, which may be appreciated best at the apex, is pathologic.

Listen for murmurs (innocent and pathologic) and any other adventitious sound (clicks or rubs). The three innocent murmurs commonly heard beginning in the toddler age group through school-age were discussed in the previous chapter.

❓ Do you remember what the innocent murmurs are, and what their characteristics are? I'll remind you of their names: Still's murmur, Venous hum, and Carotid bruit. If you don't remember their descriptions, look back in the toddler chapter. They are sometimes first heard during middle childhood.

There is a fourth innocent murmur which you may first hear in school age children. This is called a **pulmonary flow murmur.** This is a systolic ejection murmur which is loudest at the upper left sternal border, especially in the recumbent patient. In fact, it may disappear completely when the child is sitting up. This is a high-pitched murmur which may be soft or harsh; the intensity may vary from a grade I to III. S1 and S2 are normal; there are no clicks or palpatory abnormalities.

Listen over the anterior and posterior lung fields. Count respiratory rate and observe for increased respiratory effort.

❓ What are you looking for? That's right, increased rate, retraction, and nasal flaring.

Listen for adequacy of aeration and for adventitious sounds. The school-age child can cooperate by "breathing big." You will need to demonstrate this for her. When you demonstrate this, make sure you breathe with your mouth wide open (and remind your patient do to the same). Her excursion will be much larger if she doesn't breath through her nose.

Ask her to lie down. Complete your auscultation. Perform a breast exam. If you are using a drape, draw it up to cover the legs and abdomen, so that only the chest is exposed while you examine the chest.

Breasts

Breast palpation should always be performed as part of the routine or "full" physical exam. While breast palpation is never a comfortable procedure for the adolescent, introduction of this at the beginning of puberty might serve, by familiarization, to lower the adolescent's anxiety during future exams.

Palpate the breasts and axillae, exposing only one side at a time, as you have been taught in adults. Describe cysts or nodules, noting location, size, tenderness, fixation to overlying tissue, etc. The tender small "cyst" or "cysts" felt underneath the nipple is a **breast bud** (or buds). These are normal in both males as well as females. Don't forget to gently squeeze the nipples (tell her first what you are about to do), attempting to elicit discharge.

Abdomen

After examining the breasts, cover the chest with the gown and expose the abdomen.

Inspect for asymmetries or bulges. Auscultate for bowel sounds. The stethoscope is also a useful tool in determining the degree of abdominal tenderness, when this complaint is present. After you have listened for bowel sounds, continue to "listen" while pressing the scope first gently, and then more firmly onto the abdomen in the four quadrants and at the umbilicus. If your patient is unaware of what you are doing, you may obtain a more accurate determination of true tenderness than by palpation. You may also determine rebound tenderness by using your stethoscope. After pressing deeply, remove the stethoscope abruptly. If that maneuver is painful, then rebound tenderness (a sign of peritoneal irritation) may be present.

Palpate superficially at first, then more deeply. In an ill child check abdominal skin turgor. Most children will tense up as you begin to palpate, but true tenderness isn't present normally. The maneuvers to relax the abdomen (discussed in the toddler chapter) will be helpful in an older child as well. Some examiners prefer to begin palpation at the lower end of the abdomen and proceed upwards. Others prefer the opposite approach. The reason for the opposing camps is related to opinion about optimally palpating liver and spleen edges. Some believe that if you begin "from below" you will falsely "push up" a liver or spleen edge, and thus falsely reduce your estimation of organ size. Others believe that if you begin "from above" that you will "miss" the lower edge of either organ. To further confound the difficulty, the child with an abnormality in body habitus or intrabdominal or intrathoracic pathology (e.g., hyperexpanded lungs from asthma) may have apparent abdominal organomegaly; in this case, the vertical span of liver below the costal margin is increased; the total size of the organ is normal.

❓ You are seeing a healthy child for a routine health maintenance visit. There are no acute problems, and no history of jaundice, fatigue, or anorexia. You find that the liver edge is down 4 centimeters from the

costal margin in the right mid-clavicular line, but you are unsure as to whether or not the liver is really enlarged. What should you do? Percuss! Estimate vertical liver span in the midclavicular line. Percuss out the height of liver "dullness" above the costal margin; add to that the vertical length of liver palpated below the costal margin. In the school-age child the total vertical liver span assessed using this method should not exceed approximately 9 to 10 cm.[9] If total liver span is normal, carefully reexamine the chest and lungs and rest of the abdomen listening for adventitious sounds and examining for thoracic or intrabdominal pathology.

The preadolescent can cooperate enough to "take a big breath" while you palpate; this will enhance your ability to feel liver and spleen edges as they flip up over your fingertips during inspiration or pass downwards over your fingertips during expiration. You will normally encounter a firm (not hard) liver edge a few centimeters down from the costal margin in the right midclavicular line.

One method for locating a spleen tip is bimanual palpation (Figure 5.7). Stand at your patient's right side. Insert your nonpalpating hand under her back, just below her left posterior rib cage and apply gently pressure in towards the spleen. Simultaneously, with your other hand, begin gentle palpation down onto the abdomen, in the patient's right lower quadrant. Continue working (while palpating) your abdominal hand diagonally up and across the abdomen towards the left upper quadrant. You may feel a spleen tip flip up over your fingertips in an apparently healthy child. Many of these children have recently resolved viral illnesses. There are many other reasons for enlarged spleens such as hematopoietic malignancies, but in pediatrics, the vast majority are related to viral illness.

Palpate for masses. In most children you will feel a pulsating aorta on deep palpation just to the left of the umbilicus. Masses should be identified as in adults, as to location, approximate size, firmness, tender-

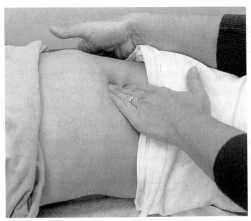

Figure 5.7. Bimanual palpation for splenomegaly.

ness, and mobility. An enlarged bladder may be palpated as a mass. This may simply be a full bladder. Ask the child if he or she needs to use the bathroom.

❓ What's the most common "mass" you may feel in a well child? Yes, the "mass" of feces in the lower colon.

Percussion of the abdomen will enable you to more accurately assess organ or mass size. Percuss if you are concerned about pathology. Assessment for shifting dullness or a fluid wave is performed in the same fashion as in the adult.

Some children with abdominal pain, (particularly those with acute pain) have definite, relatively easily identifiable, **intra-abdominal** pathology (e.g., acute appendicitis). Some, especially those with chronic, recurring symptoms, have a problem, the source of which is as easy to find as a needle in a haystack. A third group of children with abdominal pain have definite, identifiable, **extra-abdominal** pathology. There are many important diseases which fall into the latter category. Two of these, which are especially common, and may cause acute abdominal symptoms are group A beta hemolytic strep infections of the pharynx and pneumonia. I mention these to illustrate the importance of thoroughly pursuing associated symptoms in eliciting a "history of present illness" and simultaneously, to illustrate importance of performing a through physical exam. When the chief complaints are fever and abdominal pain, and your patient says "nothing else hurts," look carefully at the pharynx anyway. It might be beefy red. And, when the chief complaints are fever and abdominal pain, even if your patient isn't coughing, listen carefully to the lungs; don't be too shocked to hear crackles. If your patient is uncooperative or uncomfortable, you'll be tempted to abbreviate the encounter. You've heard this before; make a conscious effort to avoid omissions, especially under these circumstances.

Genitalia

Announce to your patient what you are about to do. Tell the child that you are going to check to see that everything looks o.k. State that you will be gentle, and that it's not going to hurt at all. You may think that this is too trivial too mention. It's not. Most beginners forget to say these things. Ask your patient to pull down underpants. Palpate the inguinal regions for adenopathy and masses. Expect to find several shotty inguinal lymph nodes. Remind yourself to palpate the femoral pulse.

Female: After a quick inspection of the mons pubis, cover the lower abdomen and groin with the drape. Draw her legs up so that her heels touch the table surface and her extremities are flexed at the hips and knees. Gently separate her legs with gradual pressure on her knees. Inspect the genitalia including the labia, clitoris, urethra, vagina, and anus. Note inflammation, adhesions (labial adhesions are common in prepubertal females), lesions, and vaginal discharge. If you see erythema of the perineum, ask your patient if she takes bubble baths. This is a common nonspecific irritator. Premenarchal females may have a normal, watery, nonpurulent vaginal discharge which is not foul-smelling. Bloody, purulent, or foul-smelling vaginal discharge needs to be investigated further for infectious etiologies (Figure 5.8).

Pubic hair (Tanner 2) development be-

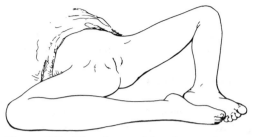

Figure 5.8. Frog-leg position for routine examination of female external genitalia. Reproduced with permission Fleisher GR, Ludwig S., eds. Textbook of pediatric emergency medicine. 2nd ed. Baltimore: Williams & Wilkins, 1988: 711.

gins between the ages of 8½ and 14, (U.S. average is 11), approximately 6 months after the onset of breast budding. The onset of puberty in females prior to age 8 in known as precocious puberty.[10] Tanner sequences and illustrations are found in the appendix.

Male: Inspect the penis, urethra, scrotum, and testes. Also, inspect the anus. The first sign of puberty in males (Tanner 2 genitalia) is testicular enlargement and scrotal skin thinning. This begins between ages 9½ and 13½ (averages = 11½). The onset of puberty in males prior to age 9 is known as precocious puberty.[10] Estimating early testicular enlargement requires experience. There are special instruments for exact measurement of testicular volume, but these are reserved for cases in which there are special concerns (e.g., suspicion of delayed onset of puberty). The prepubertal testicle is approximately 1½–2 cm. in length. Palpate the scrotum and testes. Evaluate testicular size and search for masses. The left testicle is usually slightly lower in position than the right one, but the right testicle is slightly larger. If you are unable to palpate the testes in the scrotum, attempt to milk them down. To increase pressure on the lower abdominal contents in order to locate the testes, you may need to ask your patient to sit on the examining table and cross his legs "Indian style."

If there is a history of a bulge in the groin (and you suspect a hernia), but you are unable to find it, asking your patient to strain or bear down while standing, may elicit it (making him laugh may accomplish the same thing). An inguinal hernia should be electively repaired, to avoid incarceration and strangulation.

The onset of public hair growth (genital hair Tanner stage 2) occurs between the ages of 10 to 15. It usually begins with the growth of straight, slightly pigmented hair, 6 months after the onset of testicular enlargement. Since the male growth spurt doesn't begin until genital Tanner stage 3 (and peak during stage 4), 2–2½ years after the onset of puberty, the school-age male with early signs of puberty may be reassured that the growth spurt is yet to come. The sequence of pubertal development in males is highly predictable; however, the extent of pubertal development for any one particular chronologic age is highly variable.[10]

Examine the penis and foreskin for inflammation and adhesions. The vast majority of school-age boys will have a fully retractable foreskin. If the glans cannot be fully exposed, your patient has phimosis. By this age, most cases of phimosis are no longer developmental; that is, most will require surgical release. This is necessary to prevent infection.

There may be a concern that his penis is too small. This complaint will come from his parents; he will not ask you about this spontaneously. In the slightly older adolescent, you will include a question about genital concerns during your history taking (more about this in the next chapter). A "small" penis isn't usually small in actuality. The concern usually stems from either a misunderstanding of the normal sequence of puberty (e.g., testicles enlarge before the penis elongates); or from observing a penis that is hidden within the pubic fat pad. Penile enlargement (genital Tanner stage 3) doesn't usually begin until age 10½ at the earliest (the normal range is 10½ to 14½, which is 12 to 18 months after the onset of testicular enlargement). To measure or inspect a penis for true size, retract the pubic fat pad with one hand, while you stretch the

penis to its full length with the other hand. Unless you have a real concern that there is an abnormality, you can estimate size, so as not to unduly alarm or embarrass your patient. If your inspection has raised a true concern, you will need an objective measurement. Measure the penile length with a ruler from the pubic ramus to the end of the glans. The average school age prepubertal male will have a penile length of 6 cm. (normal range is 4½ cm. to 7½ cm.).[11] In the unusual circumstance of having to actually measure the penis, if your patient is unaware of the concern, you might tell him you are just checking to see if there have been any changes of puberty yet. This isn't really a lie; (it's never appropriate to lie); it's just an additional explanation for the maneuver designed to avoid unnecessarily embarrassing him. Further discussion of puberty is found in the adolescent chapter.

When you have finished the genitalia exam, reassure your patient that "everything looks normal," (if it does), and ask him to put his underwear back on.

Lower Extremities and Back

Inspect the lower extremities including the feet. Assess bones, muscles, and joints. Note shape, size, bulk, angulation. Put joints through range of motion. Tenderness, limitation of motion, or signs of inflammation should be assessed as you have been taught in adults. Assess strength and tone.

You may choose to complete the neurodevelopment exam at this point and inspect the back afterwards. Alternatively, you may reverse this order. Choose either order and stick to it with each exam.

Ask your patient to stand and tell her that you are going to check her back for a curvature of the spine. **Scoliosis** may appear at any age during childhood, but idiopathic scoliosis most commonly presents in the preadolescent or adolescent. Because children entering the growth spurt are at risk for rapid progression of scoliosis, it is especially crucial that every late school-age child have a thorough back exam. (Figure 5.9)

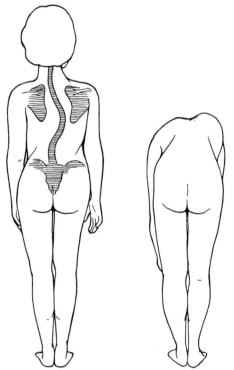

Figure 5.9. Examination for scoliosis: the back and spine are inspected when the patient is upright and bending forward from the waist. Reproduced with permission Avery ME, First LR., eds. Pediatric medicine. Baltimore: Williams & Wilkins, 1989:1283.

Make sure the shirt or gown is off. You must see the entire back.

First inspect the spine from behind. Have your patient stand with her feet together, arms at her sides, standing "as straight as possible" with her eyes looking straight ahead. Inspect the spine for lateral curvatures.

❓ What else about the spine should be noted? That's right. Anything overlying the spine (e.g., dimples, growth, hair tufts, etc.)

Palpate for tenderness. Look for symmetry of shoulders, scapulae, posterior ribs, and iliac crests. Scoliosis may be present without an obvious spinal curvature. The only sign may be asymmetric height or prominence of one of the structures listed above.

The second half of the exam for scoliosis (which also tests for flexibility of the spine) begins when you ask her to bend forward from the waist without bending her knees. Tell her to let her arms just hang at her sides and to try and bend over without twisting to one side. Inspect the spine and paraspinal contours from behind the patient; then inspect again while standing at her side. You are looking for the same findings as you did while she was standing up: straightness of spine and asymmetries of paired bilateral structures. Check carefully for asymmetry of paraspinal muscle contour and rib outline. If your patient's vertebrae are obscured by muscle or fat, a useful adjunct is a ball point pen. Feel for each vertebrae and put a mark at the site of central prominence. Then ask her to stand up. The spine will be nicely outlined.

Next, move to the patient's side and inspect for **kyphosis** or **lordosis.** Kyphosis, or "hump back," is when the spine curves out posteriorly; lordosis, or "sway back," is when the spine curves in anteriorly. There is normally a mild kyphosis of the upper back and a mild lordosis of the lumbar area. Exaggeration of either of these curves requires further investigation. Normally, on forward bending, the kyphosis appears as a smooth small curve and the lordosis disappears.

Before she returns to the examining table, ask her to walk across the room. Observe her gait. Note abnormal posturing or limp. Note angle of gait and intoeing or outoeing. Note bowlegs or knocknees.

If you examine more than a few children, sooner or later you will encounter someone with a history of **trauma to an extremity.** Regardless of whether the patient is a toddler who fell off the jungle gym or a school-age athlete who had an accident on the playing field, the basic procedure is always the same. First, try to elicit a history of exactly what happened. Second, after inquiring "where does it hurt?," look at the extremity in question before you touch it. If there is an obvious deformity, assume that there is a fracture and X-ray it. If there is no obvious deformity, compare it **visually** to the opposite extremity. Next, gently palpate at the site of tenderness and evaluate range of motion of the adjacent joints (and compare your findings to the opposite side). You may also observe the patient's ability to actively use the limb in question. Significant point tenderness or asymmetry in form or function also requires a film.

Neurologic and Development

Healthy children will cooperate for most of the neurologic maneuvers that you have already learned on adults. As you have proceeded, you have already performed some of these. Now is the time to mentally review the exam and fill in what's been left out.

Neurologically-related components of the general physical exam, especially the head, skin, spine, and a search for congenital anomalies have already been discussed.

General appearance and mental status. This includes observations of alertness, mood, cognitive skills, and language. Information about affect can be gathered by observation and by direct questioning. Ask the parent, "Do you find her to be generally happy or sad?", or "What kind of mood is she generally in?," or "Do you have any concerns about her mood or attitudes?," etc. In addition, ask your patient questions such as, "What kind of things make you happy? What makes you sad? Are you worried about anything?"

Cognitive functioning is most efficiently assessed by asking about school progress (see Explanatory notes on Cognitive Development). If there are problems with school functioning, don't neglect to ask about what types of assessments were done, and what the plans for remediation are. Remember to ask specifically what type of grades your patient gets and whether she's had to miss more than a few days of school this year. It isn't unusual for a parent to say, "She's doing o.k. in school." For some parents, this means she's getting A's; for others it means she's just passing. You should also routinely ask if she's had to repeat a grade. Some parents forget to mention this; others avoid mentioning it. Occasionally, when I'm reviewing a history with a trainee, I notice that the patient is inappropriately old for her grade. The parent told the trainee, "Things are fine in school." Without specific questions, the issue of retention just didn't come out in the history.

Age-appropriate developmental milestones are found on the history flow sheets (with explanations in the Explanatory notes section). Some of these may be assessed by history (e.g., "does she use a scissors?"). Some of this information will come out in general conversation (e.g., "does she understand the difference between right and wrong?"). Some of these must be observed by the examiner (e.g., copying an age-appropriate figure).

Cranial nerves. Assess as completely as possible. Review the cranial nerve exam and fill in the ones you've left out during your head and neck exam.

Motor. You have completed most of this. Assess bulk by observation and palpation; assess tone and strength by passive and active movements of limbs. You've observed gross motor movements when you asked your patient to walk, sit up, lie down, bend down, etc. You may observe fine motor movements as you review the manipulations of tying shoelaces and copying an age-appropriate figure.

Coordination. These observations are made while assessing large and small motor movements. The school-age child should be able to perform rapid alternating movements such as opposition of thumb to fifth finger (then thumb to each other successive finger in rapid sequence); by age 8 this should be performed within 5 seconds.

Station and Gait. Observe her station with feet together and eyes open and closed

(Romberg test). Then ask her to walk and run. Limp, clumsiness, asymmetries, posturing should be identified. Asking her to run down the hall will accentuate subtleties in posturing.

"Soft Signs". As your patient performs some of the maneuvers requested of her during the neuro-developmental assessment, watch out for "soft" neurologic signs. These are findings which would be considered normal in a younger child, but if still present in an older child, suggest neuromaturational immaturity. Some studies have demonstrated a relationship between the presence of these findings and learning difficulties. Some examples of soft signs in the school-age child include: dystonic posturing of the hands and arms while walking across the room on the heels, mirror movements of the opposite hand while performing rapid opposition movements of the thumb and forefinger, and easily observed movements of the tongue while the patient is writing.[12]

Unwanted Movements.   Observe for tremors, tics, or other involuntary movements. Within this category, tics are especially common in the school-age child and adolescent. Tics are rapid, sudden, frequent, irregularly occurring involuntary stereotypical movements or vocalizations. These repetitive movements usually involve a functionally related muscle group or groups. Tics may be simple (e.g., eye blinking, winking, coughing), or more complex (e.g., assumption of a squatting posture). The stereotypical nature of the movements is the main feature distinguishing tics from chorea.[13]

Sensory.   Children in middle childhood can cooperate for most types of formal sensory testing (if necessary). Response to light touch, pin prick, vibration, and position sense may be assessed. Formal cortical sensation testing may be performed in a manner similar to adults. These might include identifying common objects or shapes (stereognosis) or two-point discrimination.

Reflexes.   Deep tendon reflexes should be tested and graded as you have learned on adults: biceps, triceps, brachioradialis, patellar, and Achilles. You may need to distract your patient by asking her to "pull" on her fingers with her opposite hand in order to elicit reflexes. Attempt to elicit ankle clonus. A few beats of ankle clonus may be within normal limits assuming the child is not otherwise hyperflexic or does not otherwise have increased tone. The Babinski response should be absent.

Superficial reflexes (e.g., the cremasteric reflex) need only be elicited if there are concerns about the integrity of the neurologic system.

When you have finished your exam, thank your patient for her cooperation. If findings are normal, reaffirm that to her. If puberty has begun, reaffirm that everything is preceeding normally. If you are seeing an older school-age child, mention that in the future, her parent will wait in the waiting room for most of the visit. It is important to prepare her for this upcoming change in the clinical encounter.

THE PROBLEM: "CARRIE IS TIRED."

The inpatient floor is humming with activity. Your ward team is finishing rounds. The senior resident's beeper goes off, and he leaves to answer his page. Several minutes later Scott returns and calls you aside. He tells you the first admission of the day has arrived on the floor. It's your turn to take a new patient.

Dr. Bloom, a local pediatrician, has admitted a 10-year-old female (Carrie Anderson) with: fatigue and a 10-pound weight loss. She is a longstanding patient of his but rarely comes to the office for sick visits. Her last visit was six months ago, for a school physical exam. On that day she weighed 10 pounds more than she did yesterday. During her prior routine visit, only one problem surfaced, extreme parental marital discord. Yesterday, her father brought her to the doctor's office because of "falling energy level." Carrie is unable to continue to play school soccer because of fatigue. Father has noticed that she "looks a little thin" but has attributed it to "just slimming out." It was the change in activity level that prompted the office visit.

Her physical exam yesterday was within normal limits except for her weight and her affect. She appeared tired and withdrawn. Dr. Bloom wanted to schedule an outpatient evaluation, but Mr. Anderson was reluctant to agree to the multiple appointments involved. Dr. Bloom also suggested a psychiatric consultation. Again, Mr. Anderson didn't immediately consent. Dr. Bloom was more successful when he suggested an alternative plan, inpatient evaluation.

You gather your instruments and review the flow sheet for the ten-year-old's history. Having done your **preparation,** you realize that you need to inquire about temperament, peers, school, and autonomy/independence in this preadolescent-early adolescent. With her parents' history of marital discord and the knowledge that she looked withdrawn yesterday, assessing affective functioning both within the family and within the peer group will be particularly important. Your **preparation** has also reminded you that "somatic complaints" are particularly common in the preadolescent. In addition, since you know that you are unlikely to find something unexpected on physical exam, without being forewarned in the history, you realize that you need to be **very** detailed in your questioning and include a thorough review of systems. As you head toward Carrie's room, you also prepare yourself to **observe** her affect, speech, and movements carefully.

As you enter, you note that Carrie is sitting on her bed watching television. An adult male (whom you presume is Mr. Anderson) is pacing back and forth. You introduce yourself to Carrie and ask her to identify her father. Mr. Anderson tells you that he has to get back to the office. He asks you if it's o.k. to leave now.

You respond by asking him to stay for a little while so that you can obtain Carrie's medical history from him. He responds be telling you that Carrie has always been "perfectly healthy" and has never has any medical problems. She has never been hospitalized and has never taken any medications. He adds, "My wife will be in after work. There isn't much more to tell, but she can fill you in on whatever else you need to know." With that, he leans over to Carrie, and kisses her goodbye. He adds that he, too, will be back at the hospital later tonight. Carrie nods and looks back at the television. Mr. Anderson leaves for work . . . This isn't going to be easy.

You tell Carrie that you need to obtain some information from her and also perform a physical exam. She says "o.k." You ask her to turn off the television for a little while. . . . It always amazes me how many televisions remain on, as background noise on pediatric wards. If you compete for attention with a t.v., you'll lose every time. . . .

You begin by asking Carrie if she understands why she's in the hospital. She replies, "because I'm tired all the time." You tell Carrie that you are going to try and find out why she feels tired. You add that some of the questions you need to ask her may be somewhat sensitive and personal. Unless she gives you permission or unless she is in very grave physical danger, you will not share the "personal" information with her parents. "Not all the questions will be hard for you to answer, so let's start with some of the easy ones."

When interviewing the adolescent and preadolescent, it is crucial to assure confidentiality. At the same time, you must be frank with her and give her a sense of when the rare occasion might necessitate that both of you share information with her parents.

You obtain a "history of present illness" and find out Carrie is in the fifth grade. She has been playing soccer since second grade and enjoys it very much. After the winter, she began to go to practice in preparation for the spring season. She has always been the starting fullback for her team. Since practice began again, she has not been able to keep up with her teammates. She hasn't been able to run as fast as the rest of the team and has had to rest frequently. Finally, the coach called her parents and voiced his concern. It was his phone call that prompted the visit to the doctor. You ask Carrie if she has been feeling more tired otherwise. She says, "I guess so." You ask her to explain. She says, "Well, I go to bed earlier than I used to; I used to go to bed at 9 o'clock and now I go to bed at 8 o'clock."

You obtain some further information: Carrie sleeps through the night. She feels fine when she wakes up in the morning. She doesn't have any complaints of pain. She isn't short of breath. She doesn't eat a large variety of foods, but she never did. When you ask her if she eats less now than before, she replies, "maybe." You ask if she's been trying to lose weight. She answers, "no." She did notice that her clothes were looser, but most of her clothes are sweat suit type outfits and they are "big to start with." You ask Carrie if she thinks she's too thin. She replies, "a little." Her parents hadn't discussed her weight with her. You ask her to describe a typical day (including what she eats). The quantities she describes are very small. She denies vomiting (including self induced) and diarrhea. She admits that she doesn't have a bowel movement very often. It is sometimes painful for her to go to the bathroom, and sometimes her stools are "like pebbles." They are very dark brown. She has never seen any blood in her stools.

Carrie does very well in school.

❓ Ask what her grades are!

She gets mostly A's. She likes school.

❓ Ask specifically if her grades have changed at all. She replies that lately she has gotten mostly B's, and she did get one C on a math test last week. (Even with good students it is very important to ask about recent grade changes.)

She has never changed schools.

Carrie has a best friend named Debbie. She has other friends that she sees after school. She lists 4 names for you. She doesn't do any other specific activities after school except for homework and seeing friends.

As you talk you find Carrie to be a friendly and quiet child. She doesn't seem sad to you, but she does look a little pale and tired.

You ask her to tell you about her living situation, "Who lives in the house with you?" She replies that she lives with her mom and dad. They have always lived in the same house. She has her own room. She is an only child. Both parents work full time. Her father works for an insurance company, and her mother works for a computer company. Carrie has a key to the house and lets herself in after school. She stays home alone until her parents get home from work at 6 o'clock. Her mom usually makes dinner, and she and her mom eat together. Her dad usually doesn't get home until "much later."

You begin to probe a little deeper and find out that her parents "don't get along at all." They often "yell a lot" and talk about divorce. When you ask Carrie if she worries about that, she quietly replies, "Yes, sometimes." You ask if there are other things that worry her. She replies, "not really." She feels she can talk to her mom about problems ("not my dad") but doesn't very often. When you probe her about her father, she says, "He's not around much. He's busy and worried a lot. . . . My mom's pretty busy, too." You then search for other depressive symptoms. She says

that sometimes she feels sad, especially when her parents argue. She wishes her mom was home when she arrived from school. But often, soccer practice, dates with friends, and homework keep her busy. She denies feeling worried, unhappy, or nervous "most of the time."

Since she has been able to talk about the stress at home, you continue to ask some of the more sensitive questions. She denies experience with drugs, alcohol, cigarettes. She is just beginning to get interested in "boys" but hasn't had any experience with sexual activity. She denies sexual or physical abuse. She has discussed sex "a little" with her mom.

You attempt to elicit a past medical history. Carrie is unable to supply the details but essentially confirms what her father told you earlier. Carrie doesn't know the details of family history. Further review of systems is negative. You decide to call Mrs. Anderson later to obtain further history.

With the information you have obtained thus far, you begin to formulate a problem list: *a*) fatigue, *b*) weight loss, *c*) recent school performance deterioration, *d*) parental marital discord, *e*) constipation. This is just from the history! Do these problems all tie in together to one larger problem for Carrie (e.g., depression or eating disorder)? They certainly could. But this could also be a child with a physical problem who also comes from a troubled household. You need more information.

It's time to examine Carrie. You draw the curtain around her bed and ask her to put on a gown. You tell her you'll be right back to examine her.

While you are waiting, you review her measurements. She is 10½ years old. She weighs: 55 lbs. and is 56 in. tall.

❓ What does this information tell you? (Stop and plot in right now, before you examine her!) By *comparing a child's findings to her peers,* you find that she is in the 5th % for weight and the 50th % for height. What else should you plot? Right, her weight six months ago. *By evaluating her progress over time,* her thinness becomes even more dramatic (and worrisome).

You step back into the room and begin your exam. Since Carrie is old enough to cooperate you decide on a "head to toe" order. Her HEENT exam does not reveal any abnormalities.

❓ Did you wash your hands? Did you check her vital signs? On admission, these are recorded by the nursing staff. You arrived just after Carrie did. The nursing staff hasn't yet had the opportunity to "admit" her yet. You might as well check them yourself.

B.P. 90/50
H.R. 100
R.R. 18
Temp. 97.8 oral

❓ Anything abnormal about those vital signs? Her heart rate is a little fast. It may be fast because she's anxious. There are pathologic causes too. Check it again towards the end of the exam.

Back to the exam. You ask her to slip off the top of her gown so that you can perform her cardiothoracic exam. Her ribs show; she is **very** thin. Her neck (including thyroid) is normal. Her skin and upper extremities appear normal, although she does look a little pale. Go back and pull down her lower lids. Her palpebral conjunctival vessels are pale (Anemia?). Her thorax, heart, and lungs are normal. Her breasts are Tanner 2.

❓ What does Tanner 2 breasts mean? Yes, she has breast buds; she has entered puberty.

You ask her to replace her gown and lie down so that you can examine her abdomen. Inspection reveals a thin abdomen with normal turgor. Auscultation reveals occasional tinkling bowel sounds. Palpation reveals some moderate tenderness (without rebound) to deep palpation in the epigastrium. You ask her again about abdominal pain. She tells you that sometimes her belly hurts "right there." You ask her if it hurts at any particular time of the day and she replies that she doesn't think so. Then you ask if it ever hurts before or after she eats. She says that sometimes it hurts if "I eat too much," but she can't specify if it's related to any particular kinds of foods, and she can't tell you much about its frequency. The pain seems to go away on its own, and nothing in particular makes it better or worse. You also find some small, mobile masses in her left lower quadrant (presumably stool). She can't remember when she had her last bowel movement. Her liver and spleen are not enlarged and there are no

other masses. She has no pubic hair. Her external genitalia are normal.

Her pulses and lymph nodes are normal as are her lower extremities. You ask her to stand and inspect her back. There is no scoliosis, kyphosis, or lordosis.

Her gait is normal. She sits down on the bed and you mentally review the neurologic exam and prepare to fill in the maneuvers you've left out.

General appearance and mental status: She is alert and oriented. She's less anxious than she was when you introduced yourself. She giggles at your jokes. She denies suicidal ideation but does admit to feeling tired. She performs the maneuvers in the "developmental milestones" section without difficulty. The rest of the neurologic exam including: cranial nerves, motor, coordination, sensory and reflexes, is within normal limits.

You allow her to return to the television. A phone call to Mrs. Anderson confirms that her past medical history is unremarkable. Her family history is a bit more informative. Mr. Anderson is 40. He has peptic ulcer disease and takes various medicines which relieve his symptoms. He has never been hospitalized. Mrs. Anderson is 38 and in good health. Paternal grandparents died in a car accident one year ago. Maternal grandparents are alive and well. They live 1000 miles away and do not see their grandchild or daughter very often. Mrs. Anderson has no siblings. Mr. Anderson has two brothers who are in good health. They also live far away.

Mrs. Anderson expresses concern about the necessity for Carrie's hospitalization. She confirms that there is a lot of tension in the household. Both parents have extremely demanding jobs. She and her husband "tried counselling in the past" but, "it didn't work." She states that "we've stayed together because of Carrie." She admits that she had noticed that "Carrie looked a little thin," but because "she never lets me see her undressed anymore" she was unaware of the extent of the weight loss. You review the questions you asked Carrie earlier and glean no new information. Carrie has always been a "picky eater." She prefers breads and spaghetti. Mrs. Anderson recalls that Carrie has occasionally complained of having "a stomachache" after meals. She confesses that "because things are so hurried" she hasn't noticed a change in Carrie's eating habits. She needs to get off the phone but adds that she will be in the hospital later that evening.

You present the results of your history and

physical to your ward team. Scotty obtains a history and performs a physical on Carrie, too. He performs a rectal examination. The stool is positive for occult blood. You are both concerned about her pallor. You are impressed with the level of stress in Carrie's life imposed by her family situation. The parents seem "out of touch" with Carrie. You ask the psychiatrist to come and interview Carrie. He schedules a meeting with Carrie and also arranges to see her parents later that evening. Your other workup will begin with some screening labs such as: a complete blood count (CBC), a sedimentation rate, a urinalysis, some liver function tests, and pancreatic enzymes.

The labs are all normal, except for a mild anemia which is consistent with iron deficiency. The anemia is probably secondary to both poor eating habits and blood loss in the gastrointestinal tract. The anemia also probably explains her tachycardia. The specific source of her blood loss has yet to be explained.

The psychiatrist's impression is that Carrie feels isolated from her family and disturbed by her parents' marital discord. He does not think that she is suicidal, nor does he believe that she has a eating disorder. He suggests family counselling. The Andersons are resistant to his suggestion but consent to further sessions for Carrie during her hospitalization.

You "brainstorm" about her with the team and decide to do an upper G.I. series.

The results of this study are normal. The pieces do not yet fit together. During Carrie's hospitalization, you have asked the dietician to do calorie counts daily. The results are alarming. Carrie consumes very little. She doesn't vomit (You have had her observed). She doesn't complain. When you ask Carrie why she doesn't eat more, she replies "I feel full." You decide to ask the gastroenterologist for assistance.

The gastroenterologist performs an endoscopy procedure on Carrie. She has a duodenal ulcer. The upper G.I. series just didn't reveal it. Upper G.I. series in pediatric patients may miss as many as 50% of duodenal ulcers.[14] Bleeding from the ulcer explains her anemia. The ulcer certainly could account for her poor appetite (and resulting weight loss), abdominal pain, and abdominal tenderness. Her fatigue is secondary to poor intake and anemia. Family history is often positive in children without underlying secondary explanation for their ulcer disease. The gastroenterologist will begin Carrie on a program of rehabilitation and medicine.

What role did stress play in the pathogenesis of Carrie's ulcer? There is no way to calculate the precise contribution made by predisposition vs. psychosocial factors when etiology is multifactorial. In this case, a special procedure was required for the medical diagnosis. However, **the careful history and physical examination not only directed the physicians towards the correct procedure, but revealed the extent of Carrie's problems.** During the history, if Carrie had simply been asked some general questions about school and friends, the recent change in school performance would have been missed. If she hadn't been encouraged to answer "sensitive" questions, the parental marital discord might not have been revealed. If someone hadn't taken the time to call her mother at work and insist upon a detailed family history, the recent additional stress of Carrie's grandparents' deaths or Mr. Anderson's ulcer might not have been discussed. Careful attention to measurements of vital signs and growth parameters revealed an isolated tachycardia and a weight loss which had been ignored by the patient's own parents. Pursuing further review of systems while performing the physical exam provided a subtle but important clue to the diagnosis of Carrie's ulcer.

Carrie's parents must be convinced that a "cure" depends on more than just physical remedies. In this case, the information obtained through history and physical will support the recommendation for family counselling. What decision the Andersons will ultimately make about their marriage is unknown. However, they will need to understand how the unresolved tension in their own lives has affected their daughter. The physicians in this instance have the information they need to enlighten them. I know that when it's your turn, you'll remember Carrie and the perseverance it took to help her.

References

1. Dworkin PH, Wible KL, Sutherland MC, Humphrey N. Manual of pediatric anticipatory guidance. Morgantown, West Virginia: West Virginia University Medical Center, 1985:56.
2. American Academy of Pediatrics Committee on Pyschosocial Aspects of Child and Family Health. Guidelines for health supervision. 2nd ed. Elk Grove Village, Illinois; American Academy of Pediatrics, 1988:75.
3. Dworkin PH, Wible KL, Sutherland MC, Humphrey N. Manual of pediatric anticipatory guid-

ance. Morgantown, West Virginia: West Virginia University Medical Center, 1985:61.

4. American Academy of Pediatrics Committee on Practice and Ambulatory Medicine. Vision screening and eye examination in children. Pediatrics 1986;77:919.

5. American Academy of Pediatrics Committee on Practice and Ambulatory Medicine. Recommendations for preventive pediatric health care. In: Guidelines for health supervision. 2nd ed. Elk Grove Village, Illinois; American Academy of Pediatrics, 1988:158.

6. Tanner JM. Growth at adolescence, 2nd ed. Oxford, England: Blackwell Scientific Publications, 1962.

7. Hoekelman RA. The physical examination of infants and children. In: Bates B. A guideline to physical examination. 3rd ed. Philadelphia, Pennsylvania; J.B. Lippincott, 1983:490.

8. Engle MA. Heart sounds and murmurs in diagnosis of heart disease. Ped Ann 1981;10:21.

9. Walker WA, Mathis RK, Hepatomegaly. Pediatr Clin North Am 1975;22:933.

10. Copeland KC. Variations in normal sexual development. Pediatr Rev 1986;8:18–25.

11. McMillan JA, Stockman JA, Oski FA. The whole pediatrician catalogue, Vol. 2. Philadelphia: W.B. Saunders Co., 1979:88.

12. Dworkin PH. School failure. Pediatr Rev 1989; 10:309.

13. Golden GS. Tic disorders in childhood. Pediatr Rev 1987;8:229–234.

14. Nord KS. Peptic ulcer disease in the pediatric population. Pediatr Clin North Am 1988;35:129.

15. Schmitt BD. Preschoolers who refuse to be examined: fearful or spoiled? Am J Dis Child 1984; 138:443–446.

CHAPTER 6

Adolescent

THE ADOLESCENT HISTORY
Drugs, Sex, and Rock and Roll
Student Task

1. Obtain an adolescent history.

Throughout this text, we have spoken about many "tricks of the trade" that pediatricians use to secure cooperation of reluctant or fearful children. Many of you have had to learn new content (e.g., developmental fears) in order to **prepare** for success in encounters with younger children. The issues pertinent to the adolescent may be more familiar to you, that is, memories of your own adolescence are easier to conjure up than those of your toddler years. Nonetheless, don't skip the **preparation** step with your adolescent patient. She will be physically cooperative, but not necessarily physically comfortable. She may be verbally cooperative, but not necessarily open. You will be asking her to discuss matters that are private and sensitive. In order to put her at ease, you need to be **intimately** acquainted with the issues (theoretically **and** practically), **and** you need to be comfortable discussing them.

How do you **prepare? Review the subjects** you need to cover, e.g., "Drugs, Sex and Rock and Roll," etc.; we'll discuss the specifics in a minute. **Plan a tentative order** for topic introduction. Then, focus on the subtleties of phrasing or style by **practicing with specific questions.** I believe your preparation should include an **examination of your own experiences and value systems.** Learn to recognize how your manner of questioning will be affected by your own beliefs. Your introspection about matters such as sexuality and conflict with authority may uncover subtle prejudice. Decide what you are likely to be judgemental about and practice becoming less so. That doesn't mean you should **always** be neutral. You may choose to share your beliefs with your patient, but you don't want your opinion to be misconstrued as passing judgment or preaching.

In preparing for your interview, it will be easier to remember what to ask if you reflect on why you need to know the answers. **If your ultimate goal is to assess how well your adolescent patient is functioning, then what you really want to know is how well he or she is progressing in accomplishing the objectives of adolescence.** The **physical objectives of adolescence** have to do with progression through the Tanner stages and attainment of the other endocrinologic functions of the adult. The **psychosocial objectives of adolescence** have to do with progression towards becoming a functioning adult. That includes: achieving emotional and financial independence from one's parents, embarking upon a career and becoming a socially committed member of society, achieving a comfort level with one's own sexuality and with intimacy.[1,3] These sound fairly abstract, but they provide a context in which to place the three stages of adolescence, that is, the three stages of biopsychosocial maturation which teenagers must progress through before they can achieve the objectives stated above. The three stages of adolescence are discussed in the Explanatory notes. The stages (and therefore the pertinent issues) of adolescence are more consistent among those at the same Tanner stage than those at the same chronologic age.[2] The history flow sheets are presented in chronologic order to reflect the standards set by the American Academy of Pediatrics for clinical encounters with teenagers. As you proceed through the interview, you may need to **modify** your areas of concentration and refer to the preceding "younger" or the following "older" area of the flow sheet, if you find that your patient's issues conform to a slightly different chronologic age group. Familiarization with the three stages of adolescence will help you to understand why this **modification** of the interview might be necessary.

Now that we've discussed the theory behind the adolescent interview, let's continue your **preparation** with the content and style of the interview.

Anita Soho, age 12, has never been to the clinic before. Her family recently moved to the area. She requires a history and physical examination before starting her new school. While the office nurse weighs her and measures her, you review the adolescent flow sheet.

"Drugs, Sex, and Rock and Roll" are written across the top of the flow sheet. Note that the "12" year columns have the same headings you are accustomed to using with younger children. The "Growth and Development" section includes the familiar subheadings of Affective, Cognitive, and Physical Development. For easy reference, I've kept the columns on the flow sheet consistent with those of previous chapters. Review the specifics and read the Explanatory notes. It is perfectly all right to take the flow sheet into the examining room with you, or you may want to jot down some key phrases on a scrap of paper before you enter. If by now you are very comfortable with the flow sheet system, continue to use it. There are other ways to remember the content of the adolescent interview. Whatever mnemonic you choose, the flow sheets are there to remind you of all the pertinent content. The system that follows is really my personal favorite, although you might prefer to develop one for yourself. I'll tell you about

mine: think about "Drugs, Sex, and Rock and Roll," and what issues each word might represent.

When you think of **"Drugs"**, think of health. Health signifies: health habits (both good and bad). Ask about issues relating to positive health habits (e.g., diet, sleep, exercise, etc.). Ask about negative health habits and include discussions about: smoking, alcohol, and drugs.

When you think of **"Sex"**, think about all areas of sexuality. That includes pubertal progression (including growth rate), sex education, sexual beliefs, and experiences. For the sexually active teen (or one who might become sexually active, that includes nearly **every** teen), this will include discussion about contraception and sexually transmitted diseases.

When you think about the **"Rock"** (in Rock and Roll), think of the "Rock of Gibraltar," or the "safe harbors" of most childrens' lives, home and school (and employment when applicable). (At some time during most everyone's adolescence these "safe harbors" will be shaken up, but it's just a trick to remember these topics.)

Finally, when you think about the **"Roll"** (in Rock and Roll), think about feeling "sea-sick" (a disquieting feeling). Let this remind you of the disquieting effect adolescence can have on the patient and his family. Include discussion of peer interaction (a group of teenagers; now that's a disquieting thought in and of itself!). Peer interaction is also beneficial to the adolescent; think about the positive functions that peers serve too. Part of the "Roll" discussion should include questions about personal disquietude (e.g., feelings of sadness, loneliness, or alienation).

To round out your interval history (or complete history), add the more traditional parts of the history to your discussion of "Drugs, Sex, and Rock and Roll": general health (include review of systems and past medical history) and family history.

That's my system for remembering the basic content of the adolescent history. As we've discussed, your **preparation** also needs to include plans about **how** to phrase your questions and **when** (in what order) to introduce them.

Since this is Anita's first visit to the office, you will need to review her past medical history. It's unlikely that Anita can supply you with all of the information you'd like to know about her earlier years. You may choose to begin the history with the parent(s) present in the room. During this part of the encounter you can gather pertinent past medical history and family history. You can also ask the parent if she has any concerns about her child that she would like you to focus on. In addition, you can mention some of the topics you will be discussing during your time alone with your patient. That way, the parent will have a better idea of what will take place once she leaves the room. Some parents feel threatened when asked to leave but feel better about it if you have taken the time to familiarize them with the content of the visit. With this process, you also give the adolescent some idea of what's to come. This also reinforces the message to both patient and parent that the clinical encounter with the adolescent is an appropriate forum for discussion of less traditional medical issues. Involving the parent in this fashion also gives you the opportunity to **observe** the relationship between parent and child.

Finally, this also provides you with an opportunity to introduce the subject of confidentiality. You must make your own decisions about confidentiality. You must also keep in mind the laws of your area around this issue. This is one suggested approach: explain to the patient and parent that the discussion between adolescent and physician will remain confidential. Information is shared with the parent only with the patient's consent. The only time I break this rule is when I'm convinced that the patient is at serious risk of hurting herself or someone else. In that rare circumstance, I prefer to ask the adolescent to initiate discussion with the parent while I act as a facilitator. In those instances, the patient usually experiences relief at finally being able to share the burden of her problem with a parent or other responsible adult.

You review Anita's past medical history and family history with Anita and Mrs. Soho. Anita has been a healthy, active child and an average student in school. There is nothing worrisome in the family history.

Mrs. Soho leaves the room and you settle in to talk with Anita. **Where do you begin? You begin by asking her about subjects that she will feel most comfortable discussing** (e.g., home or school: "Rock"). Alternatively, you may begin by asking her for an update on her general health and lifestyle (e.g., routine health habits such as eating, sleeping, exercise: the "good" health habits that "Drugs" remind you of). You guess that Anita is in "early" adolescence; use the "younger" areas of the flow sheet to guide your initial questions. A discussion about home and friends may logically flow into a discussion about conflicts with authority figures and relationships with parents. A discussion about general health may lead to a discussion about the progress of puberty. **Use the opportunity to educate her, in addition to gathering history.**

Discussion of the most sensitive issues (e.g., substance abuse: the "bad" health habits that "Drugs" remind you of) or sexuality ("Sex") should take place later in the interview once you have established some rapport. Many interviewers find it easiest to inquire about sexual or drug-related activities of the adolescent's friends prior to inquiring more directly about the patient's own participation. Once a teen has revealed that friends are engaging in experimentation, she may be more willing to reveal her own involvement. Alternatively, some interviewers find it helpful to begin by using "many teens" as an example and then inquire specifically about their patient or her friends.

Suggestions for phrasing are found in the Explanatory Notes. Use your knowledge about the patient (e.g., chronologic age, pubertal status, past history, chief complaint) and your ongoing **observations** to **modify** order, phrasing and content as you go along. Review of old records will also supply information about important past history and prior Tanner staging; these should also influence the manner in which you proceed.

You may choose not to involve the parent in the manner that I have suggested. You may see the teenager first, and discuss with her whether or not you feel it would be helpful to ask her parent to join you at some point. The reason for the visit, the stage of adolescence of your patient, and the nature of her relationship with her parent, in addition to how she responds, should guide you in making this determination.

Finally, remember that **observation** should not only help you direct the interview, but it will ultimately supply crucial information in your assessment of your patient's functioning.

Adolescent Years Explanatory Notes[1,2,3,4] (Twelve Years through Sixteen Years)

Two reminders: 1. The order listed is not necessarily the order in which questions should be asked. 2. What follows are suggestions for content and phrasing within each category. There are many more questions than you will need. Pick and choose from among these depending on the particular patient and circumstances surrounding the visit.

GENERAL CARE

Let's begin with some easy questions about your typical day.

Diet

Let's talk about what you typically like to eat. Some questions might include: Do you eat breakfast? What foods do you typically eat for breakfast? lunch? dinner? What are your favorite snack foods? With whom do you eat dinner? Do you follow any specific diet? Are you satisfied with your weight?

Sleep

What time do you typically go to bed? What time do you typically get up in the morning? Do you have difficulty falling asleep or staying asleep? Is it difficult for you to get up in the morning? Do you feel tired often?

Exercise

Are there any sports or physical activities that you enjoy? If so, how often would you say you participate in these? If not, why not? Are you good at sports? Which ones in particular? Have you had any significant injuries?

Dental

Do you see a dentist on a regular basis? Do you have any dental complaints or problems?

Hobbies

What do you enjoy doing in your free time? Do you enjoy doing anything special by yourself? Is there anything special that you enjoy doing with someone in your family? What do you do when you are with your friends? Do you read in your spare time? What kinds of programs do you watch on television? How many hours each day do you watch t.v.?

You may choose to reserve discussion of safety and drugs for inclusion with discussion of peer interaction.

Safety (Risk Taking)

Would you say you wear a seat belt, some of the time, all of the time or never? If applicable: Do you have a driver's license? How well do you drive? Have you ever had a traffic accident? Are your friends good drivers? Do you worry when you are in some of your friends' cars? Have you ever been in trouble with the law?

Drugs

Some teens experiment with drinking and drugs. Do some of your friends drink? If so,

Table 6.1
History Flow Sheets: Adolescent

		"Drugs, Sex, and Rock and Roll"			
Adolescent	General Care	Growth and Development	Developmental Milestones	General Health (ROS and PMH)	Family and Psycho-Social

Twelve Years	Health Habits
	Diet
	Sleep
	Exercise
	Dental
	Hobbies
	Safety
	  risk taking
	Drugs
	  cigarette,
	  alcohol
	  drugs
	  availability
		Affective
		Temperament
		  weather
		  report
		Autonomy/
		Independence
		  challenge
		  beliefs
		  home
		  atmosphere
		Adolescence:
		  objectives
		Peer
		Interaction
		  fun/friends
		
		Cognitive
		  formal
		  operations
		  school
		
		Physical
		  sex-education
		  puberty
		  growth rate
			Jump and clap
			  × 3
			
			Draw vertical
			  lines
			
			Digit span
			6-1-9-4-7-3
			8-4-7-5-9-2
			
			Copy
			
			Tanner Staging
				Health Update
				  Somatic
				  complaints
				  self-
				  perception
				
				Immunization
				  reactions
				  contraindications
				
				Screening
				  scoliosis
				  other
				
				Habits
				Self-Exam
				  breast,
				  testicles
				
				Vision/Hearing
					Home
					Environment
					  siblings
					  major events
					
					Family Health

Fourteen Years	Health Habits
	Diet
	Sleep
	Exercise
	Dental
	Hobbies
	Safety
	  risk taking
	Drugs
	  cigarette,
	  alcohol
	  drugs
		Affective
		Temperament
		  weather
		  report
		Autonomy/
		Independence
		  conflict w/
		  authority
		  home
		  atmosphere
		Adolescence:
		  objectives
		Peer
		Interaction
		  fun/pressure/dates
		
		Cognitive
		  school
		
		Physical
		  self-perception
		  puberty
		  growth rate
		  sex education
		  sex
		    activity
		    precautions
			Tanner Staging	Health Update
				  somatic
				  complaints
				  self
				  perception
				
				Immunization
				  reactions
				  contraindications
				Screening
				  scoliosis
				  other
				
				Habits
				
				Self-exam
				  breast,
				  testicles
				
				Vision/Hearing
					Home
					Environment
					  siblings
					  major events
					
					Family Health

Table 6.1—*continued*

		"Drugs, Sex, and Rock and Roll"			
Adolescent	General Care	Growth and Development	Developmental Milestones	General Health (ROS and PMH)	Family and Psycho-Social

Sixteen Years	Health Habits
	Diet
	Sleep
	Exercise
	Dental
	Hobbies
	Safety
	  risk taking
	
	Drugs
	  cigarette,
	  alcohol,
	  drugs
		Affective
		Temperament
		  weather
		  report
		Autonomy/
		Independence
		  future
		  plans
		  job
		Adolescence
		  functional
		  adulthood?
		Peer
		Interaction
		  fun/
		    relationships
		
		Cognitive
		school,
		future plans
		
		Physical
		self
		  perception
		sex
		  activity
		  precautions
			Tanner Staging	Health Update
				  somatic
				    complaints
				  self
				    perception
				Immunization
				  reactions
				  contraindications
				Screening
				  procedures
				Habits
				Self-exam
				  breast,
				  testicles
				Vision/Hearing
					Home
					environment
					  siblings
					  major events
					
					Family Health

when and under what circumstances do they drink? Do you drink too? If so, how much and when do you drink? Do some of your friends smoke marijuana or take other drugs? What drugs do they take? Have you tried drugs too? What have you tried? If the answer is yes, then ask: How often do you take (whatever)? Do your friends smoke cigarettes? Do you smoke? How many cigarettes per day do you smoke? If any of these have been answered in the affirmative: Have you ever tried to stop? Are you interested in help to stop: drinking, taking whatever, smoking?

GROWTH AND DEVELOPMENT

The stages of adolescence are reviewed here in order to assist you in structuring your interview, particularly in the areas of affective and physical development.

Early adolescence (females: 10–13; males: 12–14) is a period during which there are enormous physical changes. Physical growth is rapid, and adult sexual development (puberty) begins. The adolescent begins to question and challenge authority and the status quo; a need to begin making his or her own decisions is demonstrated. Peer group activities center around those of the same sex. The topics for conversation among peers center around the physical manifestations of puberty; the initiation of menstruation and ejaculation increase sexual awareness. There is a lot of comparing among peers related to physical changes. The cognitive stage of concrete operations will give way to entry into formal operations and the ability to reason abstractly.[1,2]

Middle adolescence (females: 13–16; males: 14–17) is characterized by well-established puberty (with considerable variability) and with it some decreased preoccupation with body and increased allegiance to peer group. Conflict with authority (parents, teachers, law, etc.) is an important feature of midadolescence. This reflects progress towards the development of individual beliefs and self-esteem. Because this process of emancipation is still unresolved, the adolescent looks towards peers for support and a sense of belonging. Heterosexual relationships now play a major role in peer interaction.[1,2]

Late adolescence: some will have achieved this stage at 16 or 17; others not until 18 or beyond. At this stage the well-functioning adolescent's attention is focused on future: career, lifestyle, and goals. As this stage evolves, the adolescent approaches "functional adulthood," assuming more and more responsibility for herself and ultimately a mate and children. Along with this increased independence, conflicts with parents may diminish, as will the necessity for peer validation. The late adolescent becomes capable of intimate relationships as her sexual identity crystallizes. Pubertal body changes are nearly complete.[1,2]

Affective Development

Temperament and Mood. Assessment of temperament and mood is made by observation and by history. Direct questions about mood or affect are probably best asked towards the latter part of the interview. (Some other pertinent history may include questions about sleep, diet, activity, substance abuse, relationships, and risk taking.) Examples of specific questions include: What do you do best? What things would you change about yourself or your life if you could? What sorts of things make you angry? sad? worried? happiest? What do you do about it when you are feeling that way? You might then ask: Do you find yourself in one particular mood more than any other?[2]

Another Approach. To summarize, on a scale of one to ten, how happy would you say you are? Or, ask for a weather report: To summarize, can you give me a weather report about how happy you would say you are? For instance, would you say your life is mostly sunny? partly cloudy? grey? rainy?[4] If the answer is mostly negative, and you haven't explored this further, you will need to do so at this time.

Autonomy/Independence. How do you get along with the adults in your life (e.g., mom, dad, other significant adults)? Who lives at home with you? Can you confide in them? What are the rules at home? What are your responsibilities at home? What privileges are you given at home? Are the rules, privileges, and responsibilities reasonable? Can you share your problems with your parents? Do you have a job? What do you argue with your parents about? How are these problems resolved? Do you do anything special with your mom? With your dad? What other adults are important to you?[2]

The older adolescent should be asked about plans for the future including college or employment. Specific questions should be asked that obtain information about concrete steps that the adolescent has taken or plans to take towards obtaining these goals (such as applications, visits to colleges, plans for moving out of the house, plans for financial support, etc.). Inquire as to anxieties related to the future.

Adolescence. As you obtain information related to autonomy, peer interaction, puberty, and sexuality, you will be able to make some observations with the adolescent as to his progress through adolescence.

Peer Interaction. Do you have a best friend? What is his or her name? Do you have difficulty in making friends? What do you enjoy doing with your friends? Do you go out on dates? What do you do on dates? Can you confide in your friends? What do you do after school or on the weekends? The middle adolescent may be asked if he or she feels "out of step" or "in sync" with other teenagers, or she may be asked how her feelings, ideas, or values differ from other teenagers.[2] **Safety and drugs may be discussed along with peer interaction.**

Cognitive Development

School: What are you best at in school? What are you worst at? What are your grades? What do you like about school? What do you dislike about school? Do you have problems in school? What are they? Are you getting help with these problems? What type of help? Have there been any recent changes in your school performance? If so, what do you think caused this problem? Are you getting any help to overcome this problem?

Formal operations is the stage of development characterized by the ability to use hypothetical and abstract reasoning. These characteristics will ultimately allow the development of bonding to certain causes or ideals and the exchange of thoughts and feelings with peers.[1]

Physical Development

Modify the content and style of questions as you proceed, depending on the age and Tanner stage of your patient.

Puberty

Girls: Have you had any sex education? From whom? What did you talk about? Do you have worries about your development? Do you have any concerns about your appearance or your growth? Have you noticed any changes in your body, such as your breasts developing or getting hair on your vagina? How old were you when these changes began? Is one breast larger than the other? Are your breasts tender some of the time? Do you have any discharge from your vagina? If so, what is it like? For instance, is it watery or thick? Have you started your periods yet? If so, when did you start? Have you had more than one period? How often do you get your period, and how many days does it last each time? Is it regular? Do you have a lot of discomfort with your periods? If so, what do you do for the discomfort? Does it work? Do you miss any school when you have your periods? Do you use pads or tampons? How many pads or tampons do you use each day? Are you worried that you bleed too much? If you haven't gotten your period yet, are you worried about that?

Boys: Have you had any sex education? From whom? What did you talk about? Do you have any worries about your development? Do you have any concerns about your appearance or growth? Do you have any concerns about your strength? Have you noticed any changes in your body, such as your testicles getting larger, or your scrotum getting darker, or getting hair near your penis? How old were you when these changes began? If they haven't yet, are you worried about this? Have you had erections or wet dreams? Do these concern you?

Sex: We talked a lot about your friends and some of the things that you do when you get together with your friends. Are any of your friends having sexual relationships? Have you had a physical relationship with any of your friends (males or females)? What did this involve? Do you feel o.k. about this relationship? Do you feel o.k. about what you are doing or have done sexually? The reason I am interested is because sexual relationships can have a great effect on your health (e.g., pregnancy, venereal disease, and emotional wellbeing), and therefore I always ask about this when I interview an adolescent. This may be difficult for you to talk about with me. Some kids your age don't have anyone besides their friends to talk to or get information from about sex; please ask me whatever you'd like, and use me to talk about anything you are worried about.[4]

Have you ever been touched by anyone against your will or forced to do anything sexually against your will?[4]

Inquire about knowledge and experience with: pregnancy prevention and prevention of sexually transmitted diseases, including AIDS.

DEVELOPMENTAL MILESTONES

Ask the 12-year-old to jump, clap 3 times, and then land on his toes. On a piece of lined paper, ask him to draw as many vertical lines between two adjacent horizontal lines as possible. Most 12-year-olds can draw approximately 30 lines with the dominant hand within 15 seconds and, within 20 seconds with the nondominant hand. Most children can repeat a six digit span and copy the figure on the flow sheet. Tanner staging as outlined in the physical exam should be performed.

For the older adolescent, Tanner staging should be performed. School progress and athletic capabilities (in addition to the standard neurologic exam) will assess neurodevelopmental status.

GENERAL HEALTH

Obtain an interval update: include a review of systems and an update on other events in the recent past medical history (e.g., accidents, surgery) that have occurred since the previous health maintenance visit. Ask the adolescent if he thinks he is healthy. Particular attention should be paid to somatic complaints since these are common during adolescence. Complaints related to the skin, muscles and spine, pubertal development (including the size of breasts or penis), menstruation, sexually transmitted diseases, body habitus, health habits, and mood may have been explored previously. If not, review these as well.

Immunizations. If immunization(s) are scheduled, (e.g., booster DT or booster MMR), inquire about reactions and contra-indications.

Screening. Scoliosis: Do you think your back is straight? If a scoliosis screen has been performed previously, what were the results? Have there been any other recent screening tests, if so, what were the results?

Habits. Inquire about physical habits (e.g., nailbiting, tics, etc.) How does the patient feel about this? What do her parents say about it? Do peers comment about it? Have any attempts been made to extinguish

it? What method was tried and what were the results? (If applicable, does the patient want help in trying to extinguish it?)

Self Exam

Girls: Have you ever had a breast examination? Has anyone ever taught you to examine your breasts? For those at Tanner 2–3 or beyond: Today I will do a breast exam and teach you how to do one and explain when to do it.

Boys: Has anyone ever examined your testicles? Has anyone ever shown you how to do a self examination? Today I will do a testicle exam and teach you how to do this.

Vision/Hearing: Inquire as to whether or not the adolescent has any difficulty with vision or hearing. If vision or hearing was screened elsewhere, what were the results?

Family/Psycho-Social

Many of these issues have already been discussed. Attempt to obtain a "total" picture about the adolescent's home and family environment. Do not begin your questioning by assuming that the adolescent lives with both parents. Inquire instead, Who lives at home with you? If both parents do not live with the adolescent, be sure and ask about the parent(s) with whom the adolescent does not live. Do adults in the home work outside of the house? What are their occupations? Inquire about relationships with siblings and other adults with whom the adolescent lives.[4]

Inquire as to whether anything major has happened in the family since the adolescent was last interviewed, e.g., divorce, separation, marriage, significant illnesses, or deaths. Ask the adolescent if he is worried about anyone at home.

Remember to ask about the health of family members. This is a good time to review the family's cardiovascular risk profile. Inquire as to early cardiovascular events in family members. Ask if any family members have ever had a high cholesterol or triglyceride level.

Continue your interview during your

physical exam. Closure doesn't really take place until you have completed the physical too. Before you begin the physical exam, ask if the patient has any other questions for you. If not, tell him that if he thinks of any during the exam, to feel free to ask you then.

THE PHYSICAL EXAM OF THE ADOLESCENT

Student Task

1. Examine an adolescent.

The complete physical exam of the adolescent patient is performed in the classic head to toe order. You have already practiced this on adults. Why should you continue reading here and not skip to the case at the end? Because the adolescent is still developing physically, and you need to acquire the skills to monitor that development. In addition, you will need to recognize variations of normal findings and common problems in this age group.

The adolescent interview is particularly suited for **observing** your patient. By the time you are ready for the actual exam, you should have a pretty good understanding of her concerns. That awareness should be reflected in **modifying** your approach. While reading this text you have learned modification techniques designed to diffuse anxiety that you, your equipment, or procedures may generate. **Modification** in the encounter with the adolescent is also used to diffuse anxiety that may be accentuated or generated by the exam. These concerns, like those of the younger child, are developmental. The teenager is intensely aware of her body and the changes it has (or has not) undergone. The intimate nature of the physical exam is not lost on her. Your poking and prodding have the potential to magnify whatever anxieties she has about her physical appearance. **Modification** in the adolescent exam, therefore, requires diffusing anxieties about body image. Your attention should be focused on providing thorough explanation of what you are doing as you go along (and why you are doing it) and reassuring that all

is "normal" (if it is), while insuring privacy and respecting modesty.

Provide your patient with a gown and ask her to change while you step outside. When you step back in, **wash your hands.**

Measurements

Plot height and weight on the growth charts. As you know, adolescence is characterized by substantial changes in height, weight, and body proportions as well as the appearance of secondary sexual characteristics.

❓ **When are the peaks in growth rate? In girls, the growth spurt peaks on average at age 12. In boys, the growth spurt peaks on average at age 14. Remember, the growth spurt is an early pubertal event in girls and a late pubertal event in boys.**

Why is it useful to understand the relationship between growth and other pubertal events? For several reasons: It will help you to decide if all is normal or conversely, if something is out of sync. Second, it will help you to predict upcoming pubertal events (e.g., menarche). Third, it empowers you with information to allay adolescent anxieties (e.g., "Am I going to grow any more?"). The expected sequence and timing of the "events" related to acquisition of secondary sexual characteristics are documented in Tanner's charts (found in the appendix). Use these liberally when deciphering adolescent progress. During your pediatrics rotations you will learn to pursue the etiologies of delayed and precocious puberty, and tall and short stature. This pathophysiology is much more easily mastered by the student who is familiar with expected patterns, timing, and variations of normal puberty.

During puberty, girls grow about 3 inches per year (totalling 9 inches) and gain about 38 pounds.[5,6] Boys grow about 4 inches per year (totalling 13 inches) and gain approximately 60 pounds.[5,6] Body proportions change as well: the width of female hips increases; the width of male shoulders increases; the male leg length exceeds the female leg length.[7]

Perhaps more troubling than an obese child, is the patient (usually an adolescent female) with anorexia nervosa. The patient with a suspicion of anorexia **must** be examined at some point without clothes on. Why? Because many of these patients "conceal" with loose-fitting clothing. Unless she is undressed you may miss how desperately thin she really is. However, I know you won't miss the possibility of this diagnosis, because you will have plotted your patient's measurements on the growth chart. When you do, you'll find that she has lost 20–25% of her normal body weight.

Skin

Observe color and turgor. Note her general state of hygiene and grooming. Note and describe rashes and birthmarks.

❓ **What should you do when you see a** *nevocellular nevus*? **Good! Ask if your patient was born with it. If the patient doesn't know the answer, ask her parent. Large nevocellular nevi are removed in stages throughout childhood. Many dermatolo-** gists elect to remove smaller lesions during adolescence.

❓ **What should you do if you see multiple** *cafe au lait spots*? **Count and measure! In the postpubertal individual, the presence of 6 or more spots which are greater than 1.5 cm. in their longest axis (vs. greater than 0.5 cm. in the prepubertal child) should arouse high suspicion for the diagnosis of neurofibromatosis.**[8]

The adolescent patient may suffer from eczema or seborrhea. The clinical pattern of eczema (atopic dermatitis) in teenagers is the "adult" pattern.

❓ **What are the infantile and childhood patterns of** *atopic dermatitis*? **Just to remind you: the infant has involvement of mostly the cheeks and extensor surfaces of the legs, and the child: the antecubital and popliteal fossae. The adult pattern returns to involve the face and neck, and may also involve the body creases. There is a more diffuse pattern with greater scaling and fewer excoriations.**[9]

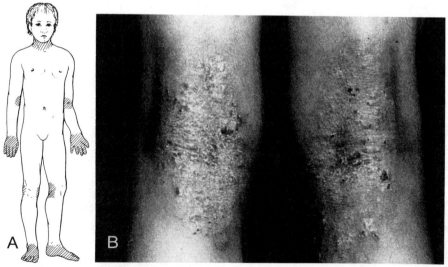

Figure 6.1. A distribution of atopic dermatitis in the adolescent: neck, flexor surfaces, (antecubital and popliteal fossae), and feet. Reproduced with permission from: Fleisher GR, Ludwig S, eds. Textbook of pediatric emergency medicine. 2nd ed. Baltimore: Williams & Wilkins, 1988:773. B, Photo: Chronic atopic dermatitis involving the popliteal fossae. Photograph courtesy of Stanley F. Glazer, M.D.

Seborrhea in the adolescent is, (like in infants) yellow, greasy, and scaly. Although it may be found anywhere on the body, it most commonly affects the scalp, eyebrows, ears, and nasolabial folds.

Another skin problem which may first present during adolescence, but not commonly prior to that, is **psoriasis** (Figure 6.2). The lesions are usually found on the scalp and/or the elbows and knees or other sites of repeated trauma. The lesions are red papules or plaques which are covered by white or silvery-colored scales; the lesion bleeds easily if the scale is lifted off. Psoriasis may affect the nails in the form of pitting, crumbling, or discoloration of the nail plate.

The "rash" that plagues nearly all teenagers at one time or another is acne. I know that every one of you can recognize **acne.** What you need to do now is to learn the names of the different lesions. This is important, because therapy should be tailored to the types of lesions present. The earliest manifestations of acne are **comedones.** The comedo is a sebaceous follicle which has been plugged off by keratin and is distended with sebum. A **whitehead, or a closed comedo**, is a small flesh-colored papule. A **blackhead, or open comedo**, (you know

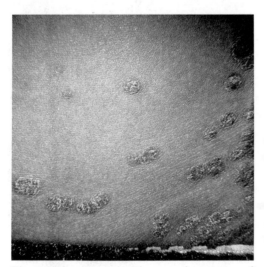

Figure 6.2. Psoriasis. Photograph courtesy of Douglas H. MacGilpin, M.D.

what that looks like) represents a distended pilosebaceous follicle whose surface opening is larger than a whitehead and whose surface cells contain pigment (not dirt). Bacterial overgrowth and subsequent inflammation may cause the follicle to rupture. The ruptured contents provoke further inflammatory response and yield the other manifestations of acne which can be classified according to depth and feel: **pustules, papules, nodules, and cysts.** Acne is almost universal in normal adolescents. Each time you examine an adolescent, practice describing lesions and distribution. Don't stop at the face: search for lesions on the neck, shoulders, back, and upper chest, too.

Superficial fungal skin infections are especially common in teenagers; these are caused by a variety of dermatophytes. The infections are named tinea, followed by the involved area of the body. You have already encountered one type of tinea: tinea capitis (tinea of the scalp). Actually, this particular tinea is really a prepubertal infection and, unlike most of the other tineas, is very uncommon after puberty. Tinea **corporis,** or ringworm, may be seen on any **body** surface. This infection also occurs quite frequently before puberty but, unlike tinea capitis, also affects teenagers. The lesion is usually dull red and ring-shaped, though the ring may be incomplete. The external border is raised and scaly with papules, vesicles, or pustules (Figure 6.3). A slowly expanding border with central clearing is characteristic.

The other common tineas are unusual prior to puberty: tinea **pedis** (athlete's foot) is a scaly rash found usually either between the toes, or on the plantar surfaces; it may, less commonly affect the dorsum of the feet (Figure 6.4). Tinea **unguim** (involving the nails of the hands or feet) may accompany tinea pedis. The distal nail becomes thickened and discolored with subungual accumulation of keratinaceous debris. Jock itch, or tinea **cruris** affects mostly males, and involves the groin and upper thigh areas excluding the scrotum. The lesion has simi-

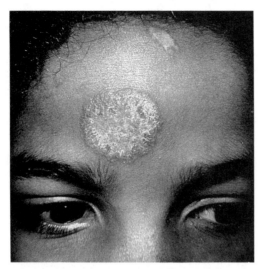

Figure 6.3. Tinea corporis. Photograph courtesy of Stanley F. Glazer, M.D.

macules with a fine scale. The macules are either lighter or darker in color than the surrounding skin; there may be coalescence of lesions to form large areas of scaly pigmentary changed skin (Figure 6.5).

Head/Hair

Assess the head for general appearance. Feel for prominences. Inspect the hair, eyebrows, and scalp for quantity, texture, pattern, and include a search for lesions and alopecia which have been mentioned earlier. Self-inflicted hair loss, or **trichotillomania**, manifests uneven bald spots and stubble of varying lengths. This may result from habitual behavior in psychologically normal individuals; it is also found in children who have significant underlying psychiatric illness.

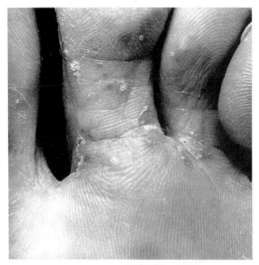

Figure 6.4. Tinea pedis. Photograph courtesy of Stanley F. Glazer, M.D.

lar characteristics to tinea corporis, with scaling and a slightly raised border.

Another common tinea (this one caused by the skin saprophyte: *Pityrosporon orbiculare*) is tinea **versicolor.** This may occur anywhere on the body but is usually encountered on the upper back and shoulders. Actually I liked the old name for the causative agent better: malassezia furfur. The presentation of versicolor is usually multiple

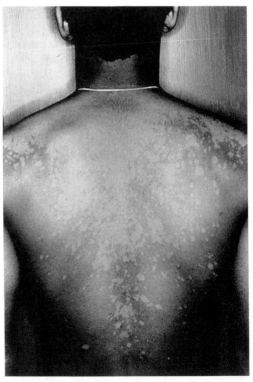

Figure 6.5. Tinea versicolor. Reproduced with permission. Hurwitz S. Clinical pediatric dermatology. Philadelphia: W. B. Saunders Co., 1981: 288. Photograph courtesy of Sidney Hurwitz, M.D.

Face

You've had ample opportunity for observation during history taking. As you begin to examine the facial structures look for confirmation of earlier impressions. Is there anything unusual or asymmetric about her facial appearance? A patient new to the particular setting you are working in should be especially scrutinized. Syndromes are not always diagnosed in early childhood. If the teen you are examining has poor growth, delayed development, or some other global problem, she may have an undiagnosed syndrome. Facial appearance may contain the initial clue to the underlying diagnosis.

Search for confirmation of your impression of her mood or affect. Is she alert and "with you," or is she distracted or disinterested. Are there signs of hostility? Are her eyes clear and bright, or dull and distant?

The sinuses are all fully aerated by adolescence. The adolescent with sinusitis may have headache, cough, fever, facial or dental pain, lid swelling, purulent nasal or postnasal discharge, or halitosis. Palpation or percussion over the maxillary or frontal sinuses may produce pain, and there may be periorbital swelling. Transillumination of the sinuses (frontal, maxillary) is only feasible beginning in adolescence because prior to that age the soft tissues and skull bones are too thick. Sinus transillumination is only helpful if light transmission is normal or absent. Gradations in between are too subjective and subtle to be useful. Transilluminate in a darkened room. One method to **transilluminate the maxillary sinuses** is to place the tip of a bright light against the middle of the inferior orbital rim. Ask the patient to open her mouth. Assess light transmission through the hard palate, excluding that through the alveolar ridges. To **transilluminate the frontal sinuses,** place the light just below the medial border of the supraorbital ridge and assess the symmetry of the transmitted "blush" bilaterally.[10] At-tempt these procedures on healthy adolescents to learn what normal transillumination looks like.

Eyes

Continue to perform the same procedures you have practiced on the younger child. Screen vision both subjectively (by asking about it) and objectively. Adolescence is a high risk period for development of myopia or nearsightedness. If vision is objectively normal up to age 16, and there are no visually related complaints, you may screen subjectively at this age.[11]

When you evert the lower lid, to check for pallor of vessels, look for "cobblestoning" or flat bumps on the palpebral conjunctivae seen in chronic allergic conjunctivitis. The eyes are usually itchy and infected; there may also be diffuse swelling of the palpebral conjunctivae (chemosis) and a stringy exudate.

Most adolescents cooperate for the fundus examination. Examine the fundus as you would in an adult. Visual fields may be assessed in the traditional manner; this is usually performed in teenagers only when there are visual or neurologic concerns.

Ears

Inspect the external ear and feel behind the ear. Pull back on the pinna to see if the pain of otitis externa is elicited. Inquire about complaints related to the ear and hearing. If this is a health maintenance visit, screen hearing. Screen objectively at the first adolescent visit (e.g., age 12); at ages 14 and 16, if prior screens were normal and there are no complaints referable to the ear, you may screen subjectively.[11] Perform the otoscopic exam assessing the canal and the tympanic membrane. Don't neglect to insufflate to assess drum mobility.

Nose

Check for patency and drainage. Examine the mucosa and tubinates. Allergic rhinitis is a common complaint in this age group. The nasal mucosa is pale, grey, and boggy (swollen).

❓ What are some of the other facial signs of upper respiratory tract allergy? Yes, allergic shiners, Dennie's lines, and a nasal pleat. You just finished reading about other facial signs of allergic disease (in the eyes): cobblestoning, chemosis, and stringy exudate. Cobblestoning may also be visualized on the posterior pharynx.

If the mucosa is red and friable, and your patient doesn't have a cold, you must think and ask about medication overuse, especially nasal sprays. You must also remember that cocaine may be the culprit.

Nasal polyps are more common in adolescents than in children, although they are not really all that common in this age group either. If you see a nasal polyp, the common etiologies are: infection (either of the nose and/or the sinuses); as part of an association with asthma and aspirin intolerance; and, as we mentioned earlier, cystic fibrosis.

Mouth and Pharynx

During your inspection of the anterior mouth, pay special attention to oral hygiene (e.g., tooth staining, gum swelling, and friability). Caries are more common in adolescents than in younger children. If you neglected to inquire about dental visits, do so at this time. Inspect occlusion. The second molars erupt during early adolescence (12–13); the third molars ("wisdom teeth") erupt during late adolescence (17–21).

Inspect the palate, uvula, posterior tongue, tonsils, and posterior pharynx. Pharyngitis is especially common in this age group. The vast majority of infections are caused by viruses. Group A beta hemolytic strep, Epstein Barr virus (mononucleosis), and gonorrhea are each important, specific etiologies for pharyngitis in this age group. If your patient has a sore throat, the pharynx should be inspected for the degree of tonsillar swelling and redness, the presence of exudate and palatal petechiae.

Neck

Inspect for bulges, head tilts, and thyromegaly. Evaluate range of motion. Palpate the neck for lymph node distribution and characteristics, other abnormal bulges, and thyroid characteristics.

Thyroid disease is more common in teenagers than in younger children. Before you palpate the gland, inspect it from the front of the patient and then from the side of the patient. You may be able to see an enlarged gland when you stand in front of the patient. Asymmetry of the gland may be more noticeable from the side. After inspecting it, stand behind the patient (while she sits on a chair), bring your hands around to the front of her neck to palpate it. Feel the isthmus and the lateral lobes for size, symmetry, and texture. The size of the lateral lobes of the thyroid may be compared to the size of the terminal phalanx of a child's thumb. If either lobe is larger than this, then she has thyromegaly.[12] Normal texture is soft and without nodules. While your fingers are on the isthmus, ask her to swallow: the isthmus will ride up and down under your fingers; repeat this with your fingers on the lateral lobes. These maneuvers will help you to evaluate size and identify nodules.

Thorax and Upper Extremities

Palpate pulses and check nailbeds for cyanosis and clubbing. Measure blood pressure in the arm. The adult size cuff is appropriate for the nonobese adolescent. If the adolescent is obese or a lower extremity pressure is required, use the larger "obese" cuff.

❓ What is the normal relationship of upper to lower extremity blood pressure? (Hint: That's way back in the *Measurement* section of the first chapter.) Systolic blood pressure is usually 10 to 30 degrees higher in the lower extremity. Why is this important? If a coarctation of the aorta is present, the lower extremity blood pressure may be lower than that of the upper extremity. In adolescents, it is also important to remember to check the blood pressure norms you

are using to see what reference point has been chosen for diastolic pressure. The charts in the Appendix of this text use K5 (sound disappearance) on children over age 12, not K4 (sound muffling) which are used for younger children.

Respect modesty: make sure the door is securely closed and draw the curtains, before you ask your patient to take down the upper part of her gown. If you are examining a patient of the opposite sex, (particularly a male student with a female patient), you should request a chaperone (e.g., nurse) for the next few minutes of your exam. This is for everyone's protection and comfort. Warm your hands.

Inspect clavicles, thorax, and breasts. Palpate clavicles and axillae. Axillary hair in both sexes begins to grow approximately two years after pubic hair appears. Inspect breasts for Tanner stage (see Appendix) and for symmetry and abnormalities as you would in adults. If you have any concerns, inspect the breasts in three positions: with your patient's arms at her sides, with her arms raised overhead, and with her hands pressing against her hips. In females if puberty hasn't begun by about age 13, or if it hasn't progressed during a period of two years after onset, then puberty is said to be delayed.[13] Menarche occurs approximately two years after the onset of breast budding (U.S. mean for menarche is 12.7 years).[13] Breast inspection is the perfect opportunity to introduce and teach how to perform monthly breast self-examination. Instruct her to perform inspection while standing in front of a mirror. You will palpate the breasts when your patient is supine.

Gynecomastia, or breast development in the male is a relatively common finding during puberty. It is most common during Tanner stage 4 (genitalia) with regression within 1 to 1½ years. The gynecomastia associated with puberty may be bilateral or unilateral and symmetric or asymmetric.[13] If the patient's growth and development are normal, if history does not suggest drug abuse (there are many drugs which may stimulate gynecomastia), and there are no abnormal findings on physical exam (especially those which might suggest hepatic or endocrine disorders), reassurance is called for. This is not to be confused with pseudo-gynecomastia or, the appearance of breast development that is commonly seen in obese males.

After inspection and palpation, ask your female patient to replace her gown. Assess upper extremities for bulk, tone, strength, and range of motion. You may also choose to familiarize yourself with, and use, the quick, easy to perform **Two-Minute Orthopedic Examination,** designed by the American Academy of Pediatrics for pre-sports participation physical exams. It is designed to be used along with a brief set of questions which basically include an orthopedic and neurologic review of systems and a screen for major illnesses, past and present. The screen is found in this chapter, in the section labeled **Lower Extremities and Back.** Any abnormal findings need to be evaluated in detail.

Chest pain is a relatively common complaint in adolescents. The vast majority of healthy patients with this complaint do not have underlying cardiopulmonary or gastrointestinal disease (although these systems need to be considered in the differential diagnostic process). The history should include a thorough review of systems with particular emphasis on the cardiovascular, pulmonary, gastrointestinal, and musculoskeletal systems (e.g., questions which search for symptoms of angina, hiatal hernia, musculoskeltal injuries, and exertion). One extremely common cause of chest pain is **costochondritis,** which is a musculoskeletal inflammation of one or more costo-chondral junctions, usually in the upper chest, most commonly on the left side. **The diagnosis is made by physical exam:** there is tenderness, and sometimes swelling, of the involved costochondral junction(s). Treatment is based on the inflammatory nature of the complaint and may involve application of local heat and the use of systemic antiinflammatory medication.

Cardiorespiratory

Palpate the precordium and the PMI; determine the location of the PMI and feel for thrills, heaves or lifts. To determine if there is enlargement of the right ventricle, place the heel of your hand on the sternum or parasternal region. Normally, you should not feel an impulse. If you do, this may signify right ventricular enlargement. Left ventricular enlargement may be suspected if the PMI is sustained or if it is displaced laterally and is more diffuse than normal.[14]

Auscultate for rate and rhythm. Occasional isolated (less than about 6 or 7 per minute) **premature beats** are common and are usually not abnormal, especially if these disappear with exercise. If you hear more than an occasional premature beat, further evaluation beyond physical examination (e.g., electrocardiogram) may be necessary for reassurance that those of ventricular origin are not associated with other abnormalities. Listen to S1, S2, (and S3 if present) individually and appreciate the physiologic splitting of S2.

Listen for murmurs, clicks, or rubs. Make sure you auscultate the neck and back in addition to the precordium, using both the bell and the diaphragm. If you hear a murmur, describe its characteristics in the fashion we've previously discussed. In a healthy adolescent it will probably fit the description of one of the innocent murmurs that we have discussed previously. The Still's murmur and venous hum are less common in the adolescent than in the younger child; the pulmonary flow murmur is most common and may be more easily heard in the anxious patient. Heart sounds and murmurs may sound louder than normal in the adolescent who has narrowing in the anterior-posterior dimension of the thoracic cage, without the normal mild kyphosis of the upper back (this is called the straight-back syndrome).

Recently, there has been increased recognition of mitral valve prolapse. Most adolescents with this diagnosis are asymptomatic. The cardiac findings may include either or both: a midsystolic click followed by a late systolic murmur, best heard in the upright or left lateral decubitus position. If you think you hear S1 spitting, consider that the "second component" might in fact be a click. If this clicking sound is most prominent at the apex, then you are probably hearing a mitral valve that is prolapsed. Clicks are always pathologic.

I have repeatedly reminded you about delayed or absent femoral pulses, upper extremity hypertension, and relative lower extremity hypotension in order to alert you to think about a **coarctation of the aorta.** The systolic murmur of a coarctation need not be louder than a grade 2 or 3 and may be heard along the left sternum or at the apex and significantly is also heard in the back between the scapulae. If you feel that the femoral pulses are delayed or diminished, look for evidence of collateral circulation in the adolescent. The best way to examine for collaterals is to ask the patient to lean over in the same manner as in the scoliosis examination. Palpate for collaterals around the scapulae and in the infrascapular areas and between the ribs.

Observe quiet breathing and count respiratory rate. Look for signs of increased respiratory effort. Listen over the anterior and posterior lung fields for adequacy of aeration and adventitious sounds. In the adolescent the pulmonary exam is performed in the same manner as on adults. If you suspect an abnormality, you should also remember to compare sides using: percussion, tactile (with your fingers) fremitus, and vocal (with your stethoscope) resonance with the patient repeating, "ninety nine." These maneuvers may also be attempted on the younger child, but in the adolescent, because of increased cooperation and increased chest size, abnormalities are easier to uncover.

Ask your patient to lie down. Obtain a drape and cover the lower extremities and abdomen. Repeat cardiac auscultation underneath the gown.

Breasts

You've already inspected the breasts and determined Tanner stage. Before you begin palpation, explain to your patient what you are about to do and why it is necessary. Palpate the breasts, exposing only one at a time in the same manner as you have been taught in adults, remembering to extend her ipsilateral arm over her head as you palpate each side. Don't neglect to palpate up into the axillae and squeeze the nipple. Nipple discharge is abnormal unless there has been a recent pregnancy. Normal breast tissue feels uneven and slightly granular, like the consistency of tapioca pudding.[15] A solitary lump is most likely a fibroadenoma. This has a smooth, rubbery, movable feeling. In contrast, in fibrocystic disease you will often feel tissue that has many areas of cordlike thickenings and lumps.[15] When you have finished breast palpation, teach your patient to perform her own palpation by repeating the entire procedure using her hands. If she has begun to menstruate, reinforce your earlier instruction that the best time to perform the exam is at the completion of her period, each month. If she doesn't yet have her period, suggest that she perform it at the beginning of every month.

Abdomen

Cover the chest with the gown and expose the abdomen. You should still have the lower extremities covered with the drape, so the only area of the trunk that is exposed is the abdomen. Inspect for bulges, asymmetries, and pulsations. If your patient is thin, in the absence of heart or liver disease, you may encounter normal visible pulsations in the epigastrium. Auscultate for the normal gurgling of bowel sounds and for bruits, especially for the bruit of renal artery stenosis which is heard in the flank area.

The adolescent's abdomen is generally more muscular than that of the younger child. Because of this, even though you may have a more compliant patient, palpation of the abdomen may actually be more difficult than on a younger child. Helping your patient to relax may "soften" the abdomen. Ask her to take some slow, deep breaths and place the soles of her feet on the table so that her knees and hips flex. As we've mentioned earlier, if she's ticklish, placing her hands on top of yours and requesting that she "do the pushing" may distract her. By the way, you may have been taught the opposite technique: that is, placing your hands on top of your patient's with one of your fingers overlapping. You may choose either method, but I have found the former works best for me.

Palpate superficially, then repeat with deeper palpation looking for tenderness, masses, and organomegaly. The liver edge is usually palpable; the spleen tip isn't palpable unless this organ is enlarged. The kidneys may be palpable on very deep bimanual palpation in a very cooperative patient; renal palpation isn't ordinarily performed unless there are special concerns related to this organ system.

The incidence of acute appendicitis in children peaks in the adolescent age group. If your patient has the "classic story" he will have anorexia, accompanied by initially diffuse abdominal pain focused primarily in the epigastric or periumbilical area. The pain later shifts to the right lower quadrant. He will develop a fever, nausea, and, ultimately, vomiting. When you observe him, he will prefer to lie supine with his knees flexed. After the initial stage, he will have decreased bowel sounds, voluntary guarding, generalized tenderness which is maximal in the right lower quadrant; rebound tenderness may be elicited. Late in the course, guarding becomes involuntary and the abdomen feels rigid. Practically anyone can diagnose appendicitis with this scenario. Unfortunately, there are many variations in both the history (e.g., the presence of diarrhea, vaginal discharge, or atypical location of pain) and the physical exam (e.g., minimal abdominal tenderness, with tenderness in the flank or pelvis felt only on rectal exam) which may or may not throw you off track. If your patient is a female, you may need to perform a pelvic exam, as infectious and surgical gynecologic emergencies may mimic appendicitis (and vice versa).

If you suspect intrabdominal fluid, mass, or organomegaly, percuss the abdomen. In addition, to assess for free peritoneal fluid, perform the maneuvers to detect a fluid wave or shifting dullness as you would in an adult.

Rectal examination is reserved for situations in which there is suspicion of rectal, lower abdominal, or pelvic pathology.

Palpate the inguinal regions for adenopathy and masses. Palpate the right brachial and femoral pulse simultaneously.

Genitalia

Tell your patient that you need to examine the genitals.

Female: The principal purposes of the external genital exam in the adolescent female are to monitor pubertal development and to search for vaginal and vulvar lesions and abnormal vaginal discharge. Explain what you are doing as you proceed. If you proceed slowly and cautiously, you should be able to secure cooperation of your patient. After inspecting the mons pubis, cover her lower abdomen and groin with the drape and bring her extremities into the desired position as described in the previous chapter. Compare the patient's pubic hair development to the Tanner charts and determine Tanner stage. If pubic hair is present, check for pubic lice. Inspect the labia and gently separate the labia so as to expose the clitoris, urethra, vagina. Inspect the anus.

The width of the normal clitoris should be 2 to 4 mm. If the width approaches 10 mm. (or greater), then the clitoris is enlarged or masculinized.[15] Vaginal mucosa in the pubertal female is dull and pink from the influence of estrogen, as opposed to mucosa in the prepubertal female in whom it is thin and brighter red.[15] Inspect the hymen to make sure it does not occlude the vaginal

orifice. Inspect for lesions (e.g., herpes vesicles or ulcers, or venereal warts), signs of inflammation, and vaginal discharges. Commonly, you will note: physiologic leukorrhea, which results from the influence of estrogen. This is a whitish vaginal discharge that is not associated with signs of inflammation or pain or itching. You will learn more about vaginal and pelvic examinations during various clinical rotations. A pelvic exam will be necessary if your patient is, or wishes to become, sexually active, has significant menstrual pain or irregularities, abnormal puberty, lesions of the vulva, vaginal discharge, lower abdominal or pelvic pain, or a history of in-utero exposure to diethylstilbestrol. During the latter part of adolescence, we generally recommend commencing routine pelvic examination, even in an adolescent without the aforementioned indications.

Male: The principal purposes of the genital exam in the adolescent male are to: monitor pubertal development, search for penile and scrotal lesions, penile discharges, testicular masses, hernias, hydroceles, and varicoceles. Explain what you are doing as you proceed. Inspect the penis, urethra, scrotum, testes, and anus.

Determine Tanner stages of genital and pubic hair development, using Tanner pictures for comparison. Pubic hair is inspected for quantity, texture, and distribution. Inspect for pubic lice. Genital maturity assessment includes estimation of scrotal and penile size and testicular volume (usually assessed indirectly by testicular length). The normal prepubertal testicle measures between $1\frac{1}{2}–2$ cm. A prepubertal testicle that is smaller or larger than that may be abnormal. Maximum testicular length in normal adult males is 4–5 cm.[13] Macro-orchidism (enlarged testes) in adolescents is associated with the **fragile X syndrome,** a common cause of mental retardation, particularly in males. (Other dysmorphic features include: large ears, prominent forehead, and a large jaw.) Males who haven't entered puberty by approximately age 14½ need to be evaluated for delayed puberty.[13]

After you've estimated testicular size, palpate for masses. Palpate the testicle by gently rolling it between your thumb and fingers searching for hard lumps. The normal consistency should be that of a peeled hardboiled egg.[16] Palpate for masses and hydroceles (these present like those in younger children), varicoceles ("bag of worms"), and spermatoceles as you have been taught in adults.

Inspect the penis for urethral placement, urethral discharge, and penile lesions (e.g., herpetic vesicles, syphillitic chancres, and venereal warts). If he is uncircumcised, be sure to retract the foreskin to inspect for penile lesions and to rule out phimosis.

How should you react if your patient has an erection during your exam? Don't ignore it! Explain that this isn't unusual, and results from the manipulation of the genitals.

Ask your patient to stand and examine him for inguinal and femoral hernias in the same manner you have been taught in adult males. If your patient is Tanner stage 4 genitalia or beyond, teach him how to perform a monthly testicular self-examination as recommended by the American Cancer Society: Once a month (pick the same date every month), immediately after a warm bath or shower, roll the testicle between the thumb and fingers of both hands. Point out the epididymis on the posterolateral surface of each testis (in a small percentage it will be located anteriorly).

When you have finished the genitalia exam, ask your patient to replace his underwear and reassure him that everything looks normal (if it does).

Lower Extremities and Back

Make sure that you have finished inspecting both upper and lower extremities before you ask the patient to stand. Remember to assess nails and nailbeds, as well as bones, muscles, joints, noting size, shape, bulk, and angulation. Move joints through range of motion and assess strength and tone.

Ask him to stand and examine his back. If you determine that there is a scoliosis, record the appearance of the spine (and any associated asymmetries) on paper (draw a picture). Then your findings can be used for future comparison. If there is a a scoliosis, determine if the leg lengths are equal. Leg length inequality is one cause of scoliosis. (To measure leg lengths: with the patient supine on the examining table, use a tape measure and determine the distance between the anterior superior iliac spine and the medial malleolus for each leg. Your tape measure should cross the extremity at about the level of the knee when you perform this measurement.)

Before he returns to the examining table observe his gait as he walks across the room. Note abnormal posturing or limp; note angle of gait, intoeing, outoeing, bowlegs, or knock knees.

Earlier, we mentioned the quick Two-Minute Orthopedic Examination designed for use in pre-sports participation screening. If your pediatric clinical experience includes an ambulatory rotation, you will undoubtedly see patients who desire a "check-up" for sports participation clearance. In our office, we use this as an opportunity to perform a regular health maintenance visit. For orthopedic screening, you may proceed in the traditional fashion as outlined in the various chapters. You might also want to practice using this quick screen, keeping in mind that this is merely a screening test, not a thorough evaluation. Any abnormalities should be pursued beginning with a thorough physical examination. (Table 6.2, Figure 6.6).

There are a variety of orthopedic problems to which adolescents are subject. Two knee problems in particular are so common, you need to be prepared to recognize these when you are examining adolescents: Osgood-Schlatter disease and chondromalacia patella.

Osgood-Schlatter disease is a stress injury to the patellar tendon at the site of insertion on the tibial tubercle. This occurs

Table 6.2
The Two-Minute Orthopedic Examination

Instructions	Points of Observation
Stand facing examiner	Acromioclavicular joints; general habitus
Look at ceiling, floor, over both shoulders; touch ears to shoulders	Cervical spine motion
Shrug shoulders (examiner resists)	Trapezius strength
Abduct shoulders 90° (examiner resists at 90°)	Deltoid strength
Full external rotation of arms	Shoulder motion
Flex and extend elbows	Elbow motion
Arms at sides, elbows 90° flexed; pronate and supinate wrists	Elbow and wrist motion
Spread fingers; make fist	Hand or finger motion and deformities
Tighten (contract) quadriceps; relax quadriceps	Symmetry and knee effusion; ankle effusion
"Duck walk" four steps (away from examiner with buttocks on heels)	Hip, knee, and ankle motion
Back to examiner	Shoulder symmetry, scoliosis
Knees straight, touch toes	Scoliosis, hip motion, hamstring tightness
Raise up on toes, raise heels	Calf symmetry, leg strength

Adapted with permission from: Sports medicine: health care for young athletes. 2nd ed. Elk Grove Village, Illinois: American Academy of Pediatrics, 1991:54.

in early to mid puberty, particularly in the active adolescent. This causes increasing unilateral knee pain. On physical examination, you will find a tender tibial tubercle which may be swollen. An X-ray will exclude other diagnoses. **Chondromalacia patella** is caused by an instability or maltracking of the patella which results in softening of the patellar articular cartilage. It is particularly common in the female adolescent who complains of knee pain, particularly during flexion (e.g., sitting, climbing stairs, etc.). On physical examination, the patient will complain of pain when the patella is manipulated laterally or medially with the knee in extension; the examiner may feel crepitance with this maneuver. Further evaluation with special views on X-ray may confirm the diagnosis and rule-out others.

If the adolescent, who denies trauma, develops a limp and has pain referable to the groin, upper thigh, knee, or buttock, think about pathology in the hip joint, just as you did in the toddler. The adolescent with these symptoms may have a slipped capital femoral epiphysis which is a slippage of the head of the femur off the metaphysis, usually in a posterior-medial direction. It most com-

monly affects overweight males in the period of the rising slope of the growth spurt. Physical examination may reveal limited range of motion at the hip and/or an out-toeing gait. If the diagnosis is suspected or confirmed (by X-ray and/or bone scan), referral to an orthopedic specialist is mandatory.

Neurologic and Development

The neurologic examination of the adolescent is essentially the same as the neurologic exam in adults. Mentally review the components and fill in what you've left out.

Include neurologically related components of the general physical exam, especially the head, skin, spine, and, yes, attention to congenital anomalies, even in the adolescent.

General Appearance and Mental Status. It is not necessary to perform a formal mental status examination during a routine health maintenance exam or problem visit unless there are specific concerns about neurologic or psychiatric functioning. At this point in your encounter, after a detailed adolescent history and physical, you should be able to comment about many aspects of the mental

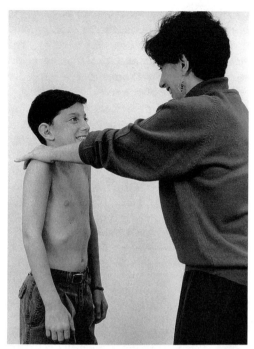

Figure 6.6. Orthopedic screening examination: to evaluate trapezius strength, the patient shrugs shoulders against the examiner's resistance.

status of your patient which include: general appearance, orientation, alertness, attention, mood, affect, behavior, and mannerisms. In addition, you have had many samples of your patient's speech and language. During your history taking, you have obtained examples of his memory as well as information about his cognitive functioning (including specific inquiries about school functioning). When you discussed his lifestyle and problems, you should have been making observations of his thought content, ability to reason, as well as his insight.

Age-appropriate developmental milestones for the 12-year-old are found on the history flow sheet (with explanations in the Explanatory notes section). For older adolescents, information about school and athletic function usually provides sufficient and appropriate information.

Cranial Nerves. Assess in the standard fashion.

Motor. For gross motor observations: review the appropriate sections in this chapter or the Orthopedic Screening Examination in the section on Lower Extremities and Back. Fine motor manipulation may be observed while the patient copies a figure or ties his shoelaces.

Coordination. These observations are made during assessment of gross and fine motor maneuvers. Cerebellar functioning may be assessed with rapid alternating movements, finger to nose, and heel-shin testing.

Station and Gait. Clumsiness, asymmetries, posturing should be identified.

Unwanted Movements. Observe for tremors, tics, or other involuntary movements (or involuntary vocalizations).

Sensory. If necessary, formal sensory testing may be performed in the adolescent. Response to light touch, pin prick, temperature, vibration, and joint position sense may be assessed. Formal cortical testing may be performed in a manner similar to adults with assessment of stereognosis (identification of common objects or shapes), two point discrimination and graphesthesia (identification of numbers or letters outlined on the skin), while the patient's eyes are closed.

Reflexes Deep tendon reflexes should be tested and graded in the same manner as you have learned on adults: biceps, triceps, brachioradialis, patellar, and Achilles. The Babinski response should be absent.

Superficial reflexes need only be elicited if there are special concerns about the integrity of the neurologic system.

At the conclusion of your exam, thank your patient for his cooperation. When findings are normal, reaffirm that fact. When puberty is progressing normally, reaffirm that in addition. Request that he change back into his street clothes while you step out of the room.

When you re-enter, summarize any additional information you want to convey or discuss. If you haven't yet asked for a summary or "weather report"[4] this is a good time to ask for one. Provide the adolescent with this additional opportunity to ask questions or bring forth other concerns. Discuss with your patient whether or not to invite parents into the room at this point and decide with him what will be discussed.

In closing, review any plans you have made to deal with problems or plans for specific future visits. In addition, review the variety of options (e.g., phone call or office visit) available to the adolescent should problems arise. If it is true, tell him that you enjoyed meeting him.

THE PROBLEM: "HE'S SO SECRETIVE. I WONDER IF HE'S ON SOMETHING."

Zachary Scott's mother has scheduled an appointment for her son to be "checked out." Mrs. Scott spoke with Ruby the outpatient nurse, earlier in the week. She complained that her son, age 14, has become "impossible to communicate with." Scott has been spending most of his free time in his room with the door closed blasting his stereo equipment. The only time he spends with his family is at meals. He barely talks to his parents or his siblings, essentially answers only direct questions, and never spontaneously offers any information. He's in 9th grade and is an average student. His parents are worried that he's "on drugs," although they have no concrete evidence of this.

Zachary and his mom arrive for their appointment. They are both sitting in the examining room when you enter. Scott looks away when you introduce yourself. When you inquire as to the purpose of their visit, Mrs. Scott says that she thinks Zach should have a "check-up." When you ask her if there are any specific concerns she would like addressed, she answers, "Just make sure everything is o.k.". She doesn't continue. When you ask Scott if there is anything specific he'd like "checked out" he shrugs his shoulders and says, "It wasn't my idea to come."

You explain the basic procedures of the adolescent visit and bring up the subject of confidentiality. Mrs. Scott looks annoyed. Zach hasn't said anything else. At this point you ask Mrs. Scott to wait in the waiting room.

❓ What did you forget to do? You forgot to *prepare* for the encounter by looking over the history flow sheet and Scott's chart. The history flow sheet and explanatory notes mention that you should discuss positive and negative health habits, conflicts with authority, peer interaction, school performance, puberty and sexual development. It also mentions interval health and family/psychosocial histories.

Review of Scott's chart reveals that he has never had any major medical problems or problems with growth and development. He has been an average (B's and C's) student. He has had a best friend in the past and has enjoyed sports, particularly basketball. Essentially, there is nothing remarkable in his previous records.

Preparation has reminded you about the important topics to discuss with this adolescent. It hasn't pointed towards any specific problems. At this stage you aren't sure whether or not Mrs. Scott has appropriate expectations for her teenager. In other words, you're wondering "who" has the problem.

You do have some evidence, gained by **observation** that there isn't a awful lot of communication between mother and son.

You observe that he is neatly and cleanly dressed. You compliment him about his "funky" sweat shirt. He smiles tentatively and tells you that he got it during a trip to the Basketball Hall of Fame. "My dad and I went last summer." This opening allows you to pursue light conversation with him about his interest in sports (and gives you an opener for further inquiry about his relationship with his father, later). Zach enjoys sports, and basketball in particular. He enjoys watching basketball games on television. He used to play on a team during junior high, but didn't make the freshman team in high school. You comment that this must have been very disappointing for him. He shrugs his shoulders. You ask if he's thought about getting involved in intramural basketball or trying out for the team next year. He replies, "I don't know, I might." You inquire as to participation in any other sports. He says, "I don't really like any other sports that much."

You continue your inquiry by covering some traditionally less threatening subjects. Scott lives with his mother age 45, his father age 45, and two younger sisters ages 8 and 12. His mother is a nursery school teacher, and his father is an insurance agent. His parents are happily married, and there have been no recent changes at home. His parents occasionally have a "cocktail," but "only once in a while." Zach tells you that his parents do not smoke cigarrettes and do not use drugs. He gets along with his sisters, who are "sometimes a pain," but basically "o.k.." He gets along with his mother, but feels she is "too strict." He complains, "she always wants to know what I'm doing" and "doesn't give me any space." You ask him to tell you more about what that's like. Zach replies that his mom is "always coming into my room to check up on me. She bugs me about getting my homework done. She bugs me about keeping my room clean. She always wants to know where I'm going and what I'm doing, everytime I meet my friends." "What about your dad?" "We get along o.k.." "Is there anything special that you enjoy doing with either of your parents?" "My dad and I shoot baskets a lot. Sometimes we go to basketball games." It is apparent that father and son share a common love of the sport. "Can you confide in your parents?" "If you had a real serious problem who would you talk to?" Zach replies, "I guess my dad."

You continue by asking about his friends. You ask what he and his friends do for fun. He replies that mostly they just hang out at someone's house. "Sometimes we shoot baskets or play video games." With gentle prodding, you're able to elicit some further information that confirms that Zach has some good relationships with male friends. He gets B's and a few C's at school. He is "really good" at math and "not so good" in English. He "hates" gym. When you ask "why?," he replies, "I'm not good at it." When you probe deeper, he says, "Most of the other kids are better than I am." He doesn't want to discuss it any further. You ask if entering high school has been tough for him. He replies, "not really."

You ask if any of his friends have tried drugs or alcohol. Zach tells you that a few of his friends have tried beer and once he went to a party where some "kids were smoking pot." This is one way to begin a discussion of substance abuse. "Have you ever tried alcohol or drugs?" Zach replies, "One time I had a few beers, but I got sick, so I decided not to do it again." He denies experience with drugs or cigarettes. "I'm not into it. My friends aren't either."

You decide to use the small line of questioning about sex. "Some kids your age are beginning to become interested in having a relationship involving sex. Have you had any sexual relationships? As your doctor, there may be questions I can answer. There may also be sexual issues which impact on your health that we should discuss." Zach looks embarrassed. He says: "I haven't been on a date yet." You ask if there is anyone he is interested in. He replies, "there is one girl that I sort of like, but she has a boyfriend." You pursue this line of questioning a bit further and find that "girls" occupy a large portion of conversation among Zach's friends. Their actual involvement with the opposite sex is largely just beginning. He has no actual experience. You briefly discuss peer pressures and offer the doctor's office as a source of confidential advice. You do some brief anticipatory guidance in the areas of substance abuse, contraception, and sexually transmitted disease.

"Before I examine you, there are just a few more questions I'd like to ask. During the teenage years, some kids wonder if the changes in their bodies are happening the way they're supposed to. Have you noticed that your body is beginning to change? Do you have any questions for me?" Zach replies, "Some stuff is happening." He stops. You repeat, "Is there anything that you have concerns about?" He replies, "No, I don't think so".

You ask Zach to summarize by giving you a "weather report" about his life.[4] "How would you generally describe your life? For example, would you say it's sunny, or sunny with a few clouds, or rainy?" Zach replies: "Mostly sunny."

So far, you're pretty reassured. Zach sounds as if he's experiencing many of the issues pertinent to early to mid-adolescence. He has experienced a significant disappointment in the area of sports. You suspect this is a bigger issue than he's willing to admit. You wash your hands and prepare to perform Zach's physical exam.

Ruby has done his measurements and screening.

Height: 60 inches
Weight: 90 pounds
Blood Pressure: 110/70
Vision and Hearing screens normal.

Zach is seated on the examining table.

❷ What should you have done first? No, you remembered to wash your hands. *Preparation . . .* **for the physical involves plotting his measurements on the growth chart. Zach**

is in the tenth percentile for height and weight.

You perform the physical exam. The exam is normal. He is Tanner stage III for testicular enlargement and Tanner stage II for pubic hair.

❓ **What are you going to tell Zach? Hint, the answer lies in thinking about the sequencing of pubertal development. Look at the chart in the appendix. Zach is "normal" but has entered puberty a little on the late side. He is still about a year to a year and a half away from the peak of the growth spurt.**

You tell Zach that his exam is normal. You reassure him that he is developing normally but may arrive at his growth spurt a little later than some of his friends. He replies, "Later than **all** of my friends! They're all way taller than I am. I never used to be short when I was little. But now I am." You ask about his family. He replies, "My dad is really tall. No one in my family is short!" You ask Zack if this has really bothered him. "My sister is the same height I am! How do you think I feel? She's two years younger than I am. It's embarrassing. She teases me about it all the time!" This is an opportunity to do some teaching. By becoming familiar with Tanner sequencing, you've learned that the average height spurt in girls occurs almost two years before the average height spurt in boys. Since Zach entered puberty a little slower than some boys, the peak of his height spurt will occur even later. Zach is a little skeptical. You decide to pull out the Tanner charts to show him.

"Do you think that has anything to do with your not making the basketball team?" "I know that's why. The coach told me I could really shoot but that I was too short. He told me I should try again in a year or two." You tell Zach that the coach might be right. "In two years you may have caught up enough. That doesn't help change things right now, but at least you know what's likely to happen later on. I can't guarantee you'll make the team, but you still have quite a bit of growing to do." Perhaps someone else in your family grew this way too. Shall we ask your mom? How would you feel if we shared this information with her?" Zach agrees to this.

"Shall we ask her to come in now? I would like to tell her that you're healthy. Then we can ask her this question. Is there anything else you'd like to talk about before we finish?" Zach says "no," but looks relieved.

You invite Mrs. Scott back into the room. You reassure her that her son is doing fine. You discuss your findings in general terms and ask her about similar growth patterns in the family. She laughs. "My husband was exactly the same way. When he was in high school, he was shorter than all of his friends. He was a 'late bloomer'. But, boy did he catch up!" Zach looks embarrassed. You add that this is a concern of Zach's. Mrs. Scott looks surprised. "How come you didn't tell us about this?"

You allow Zach and his mom to communicate. You reinforce the positive aspects of being able to talk to one another.

You didn't need a rotation in adolescent medicine to figure out what some of Zach's concerns were. You've learned, by being a good observer, that communication between Zach and his mom wasn't optimal. You've learned how to perform a thorough adolescent history and physical exam. Therefore you've learned what to expect from "normal" progress. In this case, you've identified a "deviation" that still qualifies as being within the "normal range." Transmitting this information to your patient will be therapeutic. By practicing the skills we've reviewed here, you'll be ready to learn more about health issues and problems in the adolescent patient.

References

1. Dworkin PH, Wible KL, Sutherland MC, Humphrey N. Manual of pediatric anticipatory guidance. Morgantown, West Virginia; West Virginia University Medical Center, 1985:63a–74.
2. American Academy of Pediatrics Committee on Psychosocial Aspects of Child and Family Health. Guidelines for health supervision. 2nd ed. Elk Grove Village, Illinois: American Academy of Pediatrics, 1988:86–120.
3. Smith J, Felice M. Interviewing adolescent patients: some guidelines for the clinician. Pediatr Ann 1980;9:38–44.
4. Goldenring JM, Cohen E. Getting into adolescent heads. Contemp Pediatr 1988;July:75–90.
5. Comerci GD, Kilbourne KA, Harrison GG. Adolescent nutrition. In: Hofmann AD, Greydanus DE, eds. Adolescent medicine. 2nd ed. Norwalk, Connecticut: Appleton & Lange, 1989:431.
6. Athreya BA, Silverman BK. Pediatric physical diagnosis. Norwalk, Connecticut: Appleton-Century-Crofts, 1985:309.
7. Kaplan SL. Normal growth. In: Rudolph AM, ed.

Pediatrics. 17th ed. Norwalk, Connecticut: Appleton-Century-Crofts, 1982:93.

8. National Institutes of Health Consensus Development Conference Statement. Neurofibromatosis. U.S. Department of Health and Human Services Publications 1987;6:1–7.

9. Krafchik BR. Atopic dermatitis. Pediatr Clin North Am 1983;30:671.

10. Wald ER. Diagnosis and management of acute sinusitis. Pediatr Ann 1988;17:633–634.

11. American Academy of Pediatrics Committee on Practice and Ambulatory Medicine. Recommendations for preventive pediatric healthcare. In: Guidelines for health supervision. 2nd ed. Elk Grove Village, Illinois: American Academy of Pediatrics, 1988:158–159.

12. Mahoney CP. Differential diagnosis of goiter. Pediatr Clin North Am 1987;34:891.

13. Copeland KC. Variations in normal sexual development. Pediatr Rev 1986;8:18–25.

14. Goldfield N, Neinstein L, Wohlgelernter D. Cardiovascular evaluation of adolescents and young adults. Postgrad Med J 1966;79:111–117.

15. Emans SJH, Goldstein DP. Pediatric and adolescent gynecology. Boston: Little, Brown and Co., 1977.

16. Moss JR. Teaching adolescents testicular self-examination. Child Nurs 1988;6:5.

Comprehensive Pediatric History and Physical Examination[a]

Identifying Information: Name of patient, date of birth, sex, date of interview

The Pediatric History: Record name of historian

I **Chief Complaint (CC):** Direct quote from patient or parent if possible

II **History of Present Illness (HPI)** Narrative description of the events involving present illness or illnesses, including the relevant past medical history and review of systems

III **Past Medical History (PMH)**

  A. Prenatal, Natal, Neonatal History

    1. Prenatal:

      a. Maternal:

        (i) Age

        (ii) G (gravida status)

        (iii) P (para status)

        (iv) Ab (abortus status)

        (v) EDC (estimated date of confinement)

      b Pregnancy:

        (i) Prenatal care

        (ii) Weight gain

        (iii) Complications

        (iv) Medications

        (v) Substance abuse

    2. Labor and Delivery:

      a. Labor onset spontaneous or induced (indication for induction)

      b. Duration of labor

      c. Duration of ruptured membranes prior to delivery

      d. Meconium staining of amniotic fluid

      e. Medications during labor and delivery

      f. Vertex or breech presentation

      g. Delivery vaginal or c-section (indication for c-section)

      h. Maternal reaction to experience of labor and delivery

    3. Neonatal:

      a. Birth date, birth weight, estimated gestational age

      b. Apgar scores, condition of newborn in delivery room

      c. Resuscitation or intervention required

      d. Problems in nursery (e.g., jaundice, poor feeding) and therapy administered

      e. Hospital discharge of mother and infant, including reasons for prolongation of hospitalization of either

  B. Childhood Illnesses and Exposures:

    1. Childhood Illnesses: Age at which disease was contracted, complications, treatment (e.g., varicella, rubella)

    2. Recent Exposures: Recent exposure to contagious disease: date, nature of exposure, subsequent signs and symptoms

    3. Travel, Pets: Travel to other locations; animal exposures

  C. Immunizations and Reactions: Dates of all immunizations; if reac-

---

[a]Appendix 1. has been adapted with permission from Algranati PS. Pediatric clinical encounter. In: Willms JL, Lewis J. Introduction to clinical medicine. Baltimore: Williams & Wilkins, 1991:121–158.

tions indicate timing of reaction; describe signs and symptoms (be specific, e.g., if fever after DTP, record specific temperature, etc. if information is available)

D. **Medications:** Current (or recent) medications (include over the counter medicines); dosage, frequency, duration of therapy, indications, and reactions

E. **Allergies:**
1. **Medication allergies:** Name of medication, signs, symptoms, and timing of reaction, diagnosis of allergy made by whom?
2. **Other allergies:** (e.g., seasonal rhinitis): signs and symptoms, timing and therapy

F. **Injuries:** (Include ingestions, burns): Date, circumstances surrounding event, therapy, complications, sequelae

G. **Hospitalizations, Surgery, and Transfusions:** Date, indications, therapy, complications, sequelae

H. **Prior Screening Results:** (e.g., hearing, vision, newborn screens, hematocrit, special screens, etc.) Date, results, recommendations

I. **Nutrition:**
1. **Infant feeding history:** Breast feeding, formula feeding, introduction of solids) include timing, problems, satisfaction
2. **Childhood eating history:** Likes, dislikes, actual diet, concerns about weight and attempts to change weight

J. **Growth and Development:**
1. **Developmental Milestones:** Present age and level of functioning should determine extent of questioning. List age/dates of attainment of major developmental milestones, such as age at which child: lifted head from prone position, rolled over, sat alone, pulled to stand, walked alone, held cup or spoon,

smiled, babbled, said first words, said two-word phrases, talked in sentences, dressed alone, tied shoelaces, skipped. Parental concerns re attainment of milestones?
2. **Growth and motor development:** Infant and childhood growth patterns: concerns re growth rate, motor development, progress of puberty; specific measurements may be recorded if available.

IV **Review of Systems:** Review of systems is tailored to the purpose of the visit. Ask a few global questions in each system; pursue areas of concern in further detail. Below are some representative areas to explore.

A. **General:** Weight, appetite, diet, activity level, energy level, sleep patterns, fever, drinking habits, heat and cold tolerance. Days of missed school, growth concerns

B. **Skin:** Rash, birthmark, acquired lesions. Color change, pallor, swelling, bruising, bleeding, itching. Hair or nail problems

C. **Head:** Headache, dizziness, trauma, abnormal size or shape

D. **Eyes:** Vision problem, irritation, crossed eyes

E. **Ears:** Hearing problem, infection(s), ringing in ears, dizziness

F. **Nose:** Drainage, irritation, bleeding, sinus problem

G. **Mouth and Throat:** Sore throat, dental or gum problems, speech problem, hoarseness, snoring

H. **Lymphatics:** Enlarged or painful lymph nodes

I. **Neck:** Thyroid problem, neck mass, wryneck

J. **Breasts:** Masses, asymmetry, pain, nipple discharge

K. **Respiratory:** Difficulty breathing, cough, wheeze, frequent colds, exercise intolerance, pulmonary infections, cough-up blood

L. **Cardiovascular:** Heart murmur, heart abnormality, high blood pressure, chest pain, palpitations, blue skin, edema

M. **Gastrointestinal:** Abdominal pain, nausea, vomiting, diarrhea, constipation, soiling, colic, food intolerance, difficulty swallowing, hernia, jaundice, bloody or tarry stools, vomit blood, hepatitis

N. **Urinary:** Pain, frequency, urgency, voiding large amounts, difficulty voiding, blood in urine, infection, bedwetting

O. **Genital:**
   1. **Male:** Hernia, undescended testes, hypospadius, testicular pain or swelling; adolescent: age at onset of puberty, nocturnal emissions, penile discharge or burning, sexually transmitted diseases, sexual activity and contraception, involvement in pregnancy, sexual concerns
   2. **Female:** Vaginal abnormality, hernia, vaginal discharge or irritation; adolescent: age at onset of puberty, menarche (age at onset, nature of cycle, excessive pain, bleeding, (LMP), sexually transmitted diseases, pregnancies, sexual activity and contraception, sexual concerns

P. **Musculoskeletal:** Pain or swelling in joints, muscles or bones. Congenital deformities, sports injuries, scoliosis, gait abnormalities

Q. **Neurodevelopmental:** Headache, seizures, personality changes, fainting, numbness, tingling, abnormal movements or vocalizations (e.g., tics, tremors); difficulties with handwriting, balance or coordination; weakness, paralysis, CNS infection, delayed development, school functioning

R. **Psychiatric:** Mood, memory, behavior, hallucinations

V **Psycho-Social History:** This history seeks information about the child's lifestyle, environment, behaviorial, emotional, and cognitive functioning. Questions are tailored to the patient's age and circumstances. Parental concerns are elicited. Suggestions for topics or questions include:

A. **Affective state and development:** Describe child's mood, behavior, relationships with peers, siblings and other significant people. Topics include: temperament (e.g., "easy baby" or "difficult baby,"), adjustment to rules and discipline, use of free time, strengths, and weaknesses. For the older patient, progress through adolescence may be discussed.

B. **Cognitive development:** Previous and present intellectual functioning are explored. Topics include language development (include speech problems), school readiness, school progress, and functioning.

C. **Habits and day to day functioning:**
   1. Sleep: patterns (usual bedtime and wake up time) and difficulties (e.g., night waking or bedtime struggles)
   2. Elimination: Age of attainment of bowel and bladder control, difficulties (e.g., resistance, enuresis, encopresis)
   3. Habits: (e.g., thumbsucking, head banging, nailbiting, tics)
   4. Sexuality: Sexual awareness and experience
   5. Substance abuse: Experience with alcohol, cigarettes, or illegal drugs

D. **Household:** List household members (e.g., names, ages, occupations) and describe relationships between household members. Inquire about parent or siblings not living in household and relationship between patient and absent family members. Childcare arrangements, adequacy of financial resources, adequacy of childproofing and recent changes or problems in family or household may also be explored.

   E. **Child's self-perceptions:** The child is asked to discuss his or her own perceptions of personal strengths and weaknesses, likes and dislikes, and concerns. The older adolescent is asked if concrete plans for education or employment have been formulated.

VI **Family Health History:**
   A. **Parents:** ages, medical problems
   B. **Siblings:** ages, medical problems
   C. **Grandparents:** living? ages, medical problems, cause of death
   D. **Family history of:** inherited diseases or diseases that "run" in the family, infant or childhood deaths, congenital anomalies, early cardiovascular deaths, lipid problems, hypertension, cancer, diabetes, kidney disease, mental illness, alcohol or drug abuse, AIDS, consanguinity, TB, anemia, arthritis

The Pediatric Physical Examination
I **Identifying Information**
   A. **Age:**
   B. **Sex:**
II **Measurements**
   A. **Length/Height:**
   B. **Weight:**
   C. **Head Circumference:**
   D. **Temperature:**
   E. **Heart Rate:**
   F. **Respiratory Rate:**
   G. **Blood Pressure:**
III **Observations and Findings:**
   A. **General Appearance:** Describe appearance as well or sick, state of overall alertness, degree of irritability or consolability, degree of cooperation, overall state of development, obvious dysmorphic features, nutritional status, hygiene; observations of parent-child interaction (e.g., verbal or physical interaction observed by examiner)

   B. **Skin and Nails:** Color, turgor, texture. Rash, birthmark, lesion, bruise, depigmentation. Nail abnormalities
   C. **Hair:** Quantity, texture, distribution, scalp lesion
   D. **Head:** Shape, contour, swelling. Fontanelle size, suture approximation, cranial bruit
   E. **Face:** Facial expression, symmetry of structures, unusual aspect of appearance. Facial tenderness, sinus transillumination
   F. **Eyes:** Overall shape, symmetry and size, inflammation. Lid swelling or ptosis. Pupillary size, shape, reaction to light and accommodation. Inspection of sclerae, conjunctivae, irises. Corneal light reflex. Retina: red reflex, disc margins, macula, background and vessels. Epicanthal folds. Vision, extraocular muscle movement and coordination, alternate cover test. Nystagmus. Corneal reflex, visual fields
   G. **Ears:** External: overall size, placement, shape. External lesions, canal tenderness, drainage. Tympanic membrane: color, translucency, contour, opacities, landmarks, light reflex, visible fluid, mobility. Hearing and vestibular function; pre- and post-auricular adenopathy
   H. **Nose:** Size and shape; mucosa: color, drainage, bleeding, lesion; Turbinate swelling; septum deviation, perforation
   I. **Mouth and Throat:** Symmetry of smile, cry. Breath, moistness of lips, mucous membranes. Lips, gums, buccal mucosa, palate, tonsils, posterior pharynx: inspect for lesions, inflammation, abnormal contours. Tonsil size. Tongue contours, movement. Teeth: count, spacing, occlusion, caries, staining. Uvula bifid. Speech clarity, content
   J. **Neck:** Webbing, masses, tenderness. Position, range of motion, suppleness; Kernig, Brudzinski signs.

Thyroid size, nodules, tenderness. Bruit. Adenopathy: cervical (anterior, posterior chains), sublingual, submaxillary, suboccipital

K. **Thorax:** Contour, symmetry of structures, retraction Supraclavicular and axillary adenopathy, clavicle palpation

L. **Breasts:** Size, symmetry, masses, tenderness, nipple discharge, Tanner stage

M. **Lungs:** Respiratory rate, pattern. Audible cough, abnormal sounds. Tactile fremitus, percussion. Quality of aeration, adventitious sounds, vocal resonance

N. **Heart:** Heart rate, rhythm. Precordial bulge, PMI, abnormal impulse, S^1, S^2, S^2 splitting, murmur, extra sounds. Paradoxical pulse. Peripheral pulses

O. **Abdomen:** Contour, symmetry, visibility of peristalsis. Umbilicus. Diastasis, hernia. Shifting dullness. Bowel sounds, bruits. Skin turgor, tenderness, rebound, guarding, organ size, masses. Femoral pulse

P. **Genitalia:** Female: anomaly, hernia. Clitoris size. Labial prominence. Urethral opening. Vagina: mucosa color, discharge, adhesion, imperforate hymen, tags, lesions. Diaper rash, inguinal adenopathy. Tanner stage: pubic hair

Male: Penile length, lesions, chordae. Urethra location, discharge. Scrotal swelling, masses. Testicular size, location, tenderness, mass. Hernia, silk sign. Diaper rash, inguinal adenopathy. Tanner stage: pubic hair

Q. **Anus and Rectum:** Anal anomaly, patency, perineal length, lesions, fissures, prolapse. Sphincter tone, rectal tenderness. Prostate size. Diaper rash

R. **Back:** Spinal opening, dimple, overlying lesion. Symmetry of paraspinal structures. Scoliosis, kyphosis, lordosis, posture, flexibility

S. **Upper and Lower Extremities:** Anomalies, deformities. Symmetry, proportion, bulk, tone, strength, atrophy, weakness, paralysis, tenderness, inflammation; circulation. Range of motion, joint inflammation. Fingers and toes: anomalies, nodules, clubbing. Single transverse palmar crease. Station and gait: symmetry, angle of gait, posturing, limp, toe walk. Balance, Gower's sign

T. **Neurologic/Development:**
   1. Newborn: gestational age
   2. General appearance and mental status: state, affect, mood, orientation, attention, behavior, mannerisms, speech, language, cognition, thought content, memory, reasoning ability, insight, calculation. Eye contact, spontaneous movements
   3. Cranial Nerves (I–XII): Assess as completely as possible
   4. Gross motor: Bulk, strength, tone, weakness, atrophy, paralysis, symmetry
   5. Fine motor: Assess age related task ability (e.g., pincer grasp, transferring, copying figures)
   6. Coordination: Clumsiness, assess during observation of gross and fine motor movements. Finger to nose, heel to shin
   7. Station and gait: Symmetry, balance, posturing, limp, ataxia, Romberg
   8. Unwanted movements: Tics, tremors, chorea, athetosis, myoclonus, seizure
   9. Sensory: Light touch, pin prick, temperature, vibration, joint position. Cortical: stereognosis, two point discrimination, graphesthesia
   10. Reflexes: Primitive reflexes: symmetry, presence, absence.

Deep tendon reflexes, superficial reflexes, clonus, Babinski

11. Cognition: Informal assessment via inquiry re school performance. If significant concerns are identified formal testing may be indicated (e.g., WISC-R).

12. Developmental milestones: Assess via objective list of age appropriate tasks or screening instrument (e.g., Denver II). If significant delays are identified, formal testing may be indicated.

Classification of Newborns: Based on Maturity and Intrauterine Growth[a]

[a]Adapted with permission from: Lubchenco LO, Hansman C, Boyd E. Intrauterine growth in length and head circumference as estimated from live births at gestational ages from 26 to 42 weeks. Pediatrics 1966;37:403–408 and Battaglia FC, Lubchenco LO. A practical classification of newborn infants by weight and gestational age. J Pediatr 1967;71:159–163, and Bristol-Meyers U.S. Pharmaceutical and Nutritional Group, Evansville, Indiana, 47721.

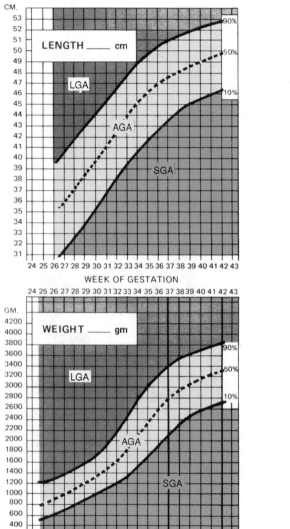

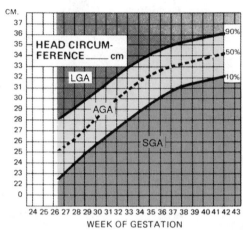

Growth Charts

BOYS: BIRTH TO 36 MONTHS
PHYSICAL GROWTH
NCHS PERCENTILES*

NAME _____ RECORD # _____

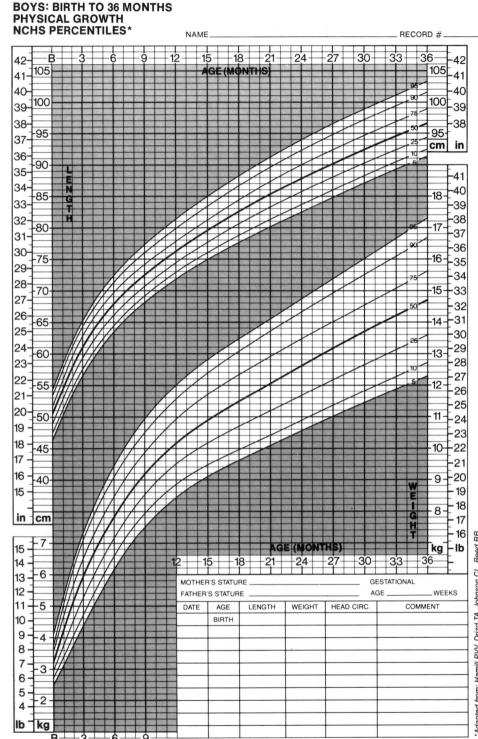

MOTHER'S STATURE _____ GESTATIONAL
FATHER'S STATURE _____ AGE _____ WEEKS

DATE	AGE	LENGTH	WEIGHT	HEAD CIRC.	COMMENT
	BIRTH				

*Adapted from: Hamill PVV, Drizd TA, Johnson CL, Reed RB, Roche AF, Moore WM: Physical growth: National Center for Health Statistics percentiles. AM J CLIN NUTR 32:607–629, 1979. Data from the Fels Longitudinal Study, Wright State University School of Medicine, Yellow Springs, Ohio.

© 1982 Ross Laboratories

GIRLS: BIRTH TO 36 MONTHS
PHYSICAL GROWTH
NCHS PERCENTILES*

NAME _____ RECORD # _____

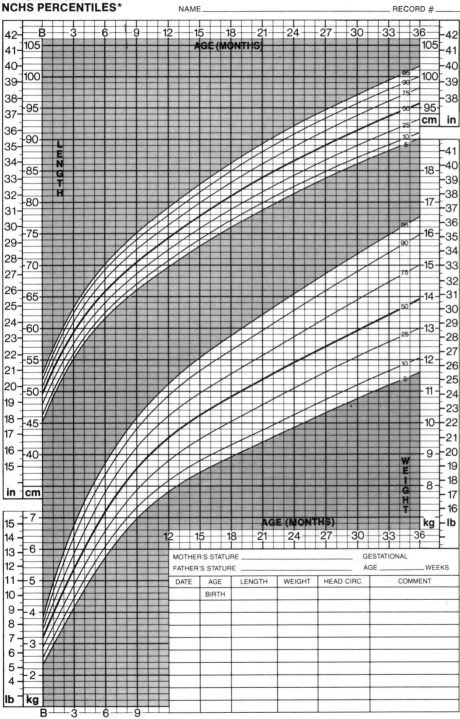

MOTHER'S STATURE _____ GESTATIONAL
FATHER'S STATURE _____ AGE _____ WEEKS

DATE	AGE	LENGTH	WEIGHT	HEAD CIRC.	COMMENT
	BIRTH				

*Adapted from: Hamill PVV, Drizd TA, Johnson CL, Reed RB, Roche AF, Moore WM: Physical growth: National Center for Health Statistics percentiles. AM J CLIN NUTR 32:607-629, 1979. Data from the Fels Longitudinal Study, Wright State University School of Medicine, Yellow Springs, Ohio.

© 1982 Ross Laboratories

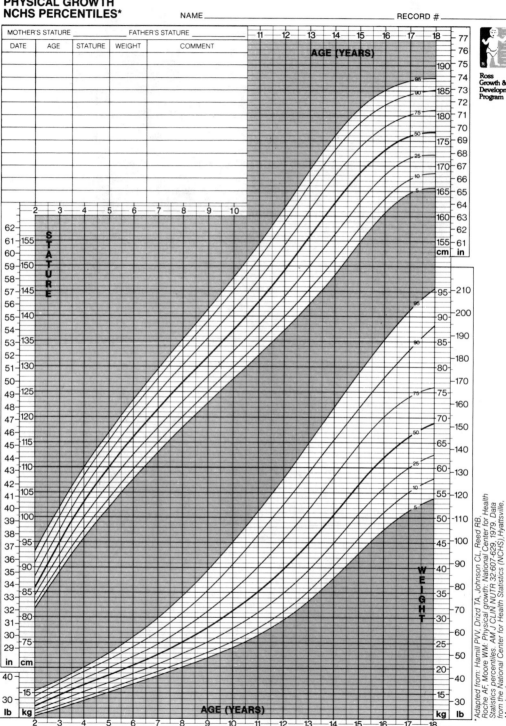

BOYS: 2 TO 18 YEARS
PHYSICAL GROWTH
NCHS PERCENTILES*

NAME _____   RECORD # _____

Ross
Growth &
Development
Program

*Adapted from: Hamill PVV, Drizd TA, Johnson CL, Reed RB, Roche AF, Moore WM. Physical growth: National Center for Health Statistics percentiles. AM J CLIN NUTR 32:607-629, 1979. Data from the National Center for Health Statistics (NCHS), Hyattsville, Maryland.

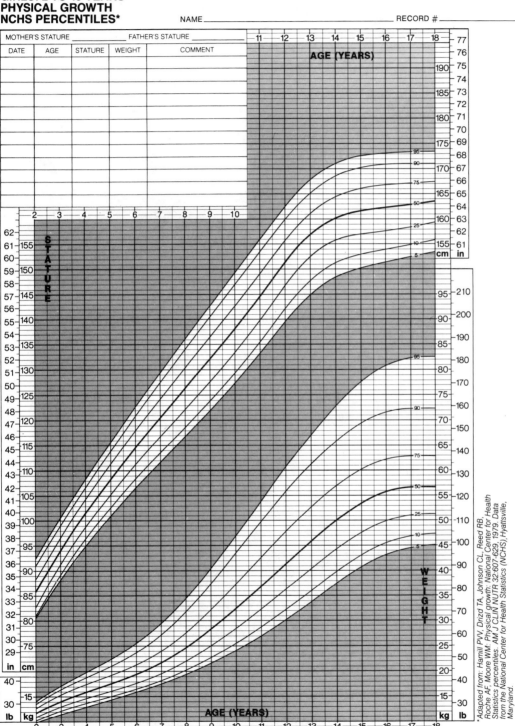

GIRLS: 2 TO 18 YEARS
PHYSICAL GROWTH
NCHS PERCENTILES*

NAME_____ RECORD #_____

Adapted from: Hamill PVV, Drizd TA, Johnson CL, Reed RB, Roche AF, Moore WM. Physical growth: National Center for Health Statistics percentiles. AM J CLIN NUTR 32:607-629, 1979. Data from the National Center for Health Statistics (NCHS), Hyattsville, Maryland.

© 1982 Ross Laboratories

Head Circumference Charts[a]

[a]Reprinted with permission from Nellhaus G. Head circumference from birth to eighteen years. Pediatrics. 1968;41:106–114.

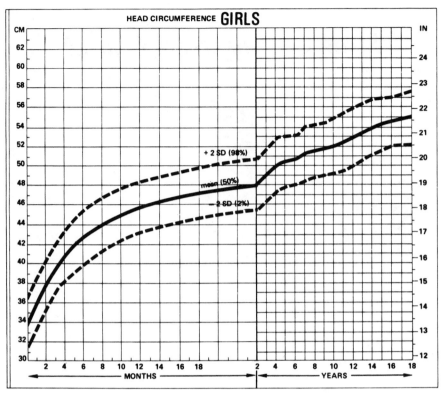

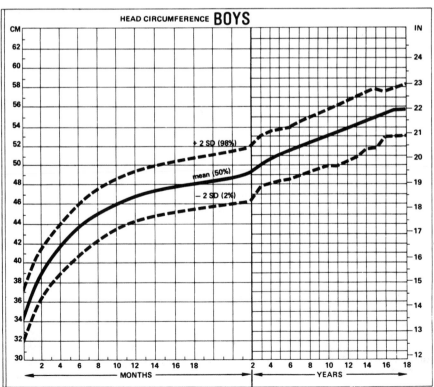

Average Heart Rates in Children at Rest[a]

Age	Average Rate	Two Standard Deviations
Birth	140	50
First month	130	45
1–6 months	130	45
6–12 months	115	40
1–2 years	110	40
2–4 years	105	35
6–10 years	95	30
10–14 years	85	30
14–18 years	82	25

[a]Reproduced with permission. Lowrey GH. Growth and development of children. 8th ed. Chicago: Year Book, 1986:246.

Normal Respiratory Rates in Children[a]

Age	Respirations per minute
Newborn	30–75
6–12 months	22–31
1–2 years	17–23
2–4 years	16–25
4–10 years	13–23
10–14 years	13–19

[a]Reproduced with permission. Cloutier MM. Pulmonary diseases. In: Dworkin PH. Pediatrics. Baltimore: John Wiley & Sons, Inc., 1987:266.

Age-Specific Percentiles of Blood Pressure Measurements[a]

[a]Reproduced with permission. Task Force on Blood Pressure Control in Children. Report of the second task force on blood pressure control in children-1987. Pediatrics. 1987;79:1–30.

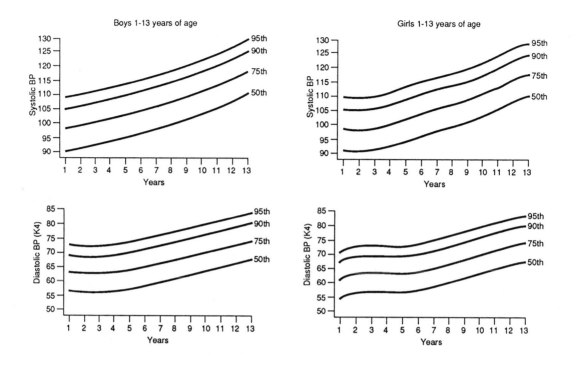

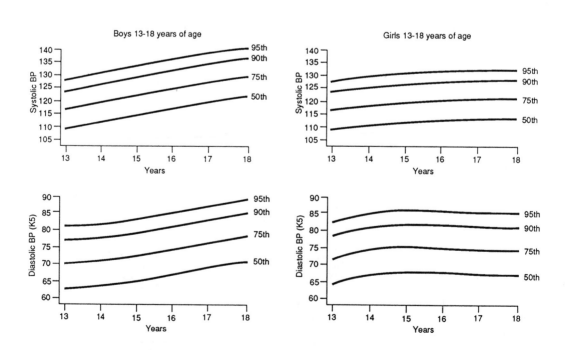

Stages of Female Breast Development[a]

---

[a]Adapted with permission from Marshall WA, Tanner JM. Variations in patterns of pubertal changes in girls. Arch Dis Child 1969;44:291–303 and Root AW. Endocrinology of puberty. 1. Normal sexual maturation. J Pediatr 1973;83:1–19. Illustrations from Fleisher GR, Ludwig S. Textbook of pediatric emergency medicine. 2nd ed. Baltimore: Williams & Wilkins, 1988:1206.

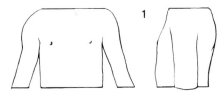

Stage 1   Prepubertal: Elevation of papilla only.

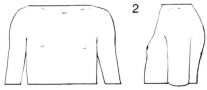

Stage 2   Breast bud: Areola widens. Elevation of a small mound of subareolar tissue and erect papilla.

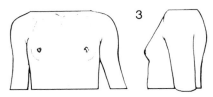

Stage 3   Continued enlargement of breast and widening of areola, but without separation of contours.

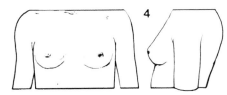

Stage 4   Areola and papilla separate from the contour of the breast forming a secondary mound.

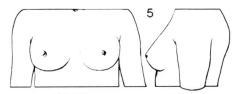

Stage 5   Mature female breast with areola and breast in same plane, erect papilla.

Stages of Female Pubic Hair Growth[a]

Stage 1   No pubic hair.

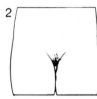

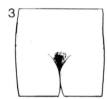

Stage 2   A sparse amount of long, somewhat pigmented hair over labia majora primarily.

Stage 3   Pubic hair darkens, coarsens and curls, and spreads sparsely over the mons pubis.

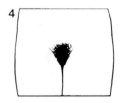

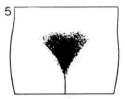

Stage 4   Abundant, coarse, adult-type hair limited to the mons pubis.

Stage 5   Adult type and quantity of hair with spread to the medial aspect of the thighs.

[a]Adapted with permission from Marshall WA, Tanner JM. Variations in patterns of pubertal changes in girls. Arch Dis Child 1969;44:291–303 and Root AW. Endocrinology of puberty. 1. Normal sexual maturation. J Pediatr 1973;83:1–19. Illustrations from Fleisher GR, Ludwig S. Textbook of pediatric emergency medicine. 2nd ed. Baltimore: Williams & Wilkins, 1988:1207.

Stages of Male Genital Development and Pubic Hair Growth[a]

Stage 1   No pubic hair.
            Genitalia are prepubertal in size.

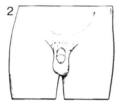

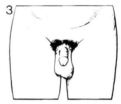

Stage 2   Sparse growth of long, slightly pigmented hair, at and lateral to base of penis.
            Testes and scrotum begin to enlarge, with pigmentation and thinning of scrotum.

Stage 3   Pubic hair darkens, coarsens and curls, at and lateral to base of penis.
            Penis lengthens and testes and scrotum further enlarge.

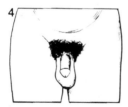

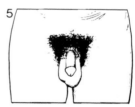

Stage 4   Abundant, coarse adult-type hair limited to the pubic region with no extension to the thighs.
            Further growth of testes and scrotum, with increased pigmentation of scrotum, and, Increase in width and length of penis.

Stage 5   Adult type and quantity of hair with spread to the medial aspects of the thighs.
            Adult size and shape of genitalia.

---

[a]Adapted with permission from Marshall WA, Tanner JM. Variations in patterns of pubertal changes in boys. Arch Dis Child 1970;45:13–23 and Root AW. Endocrinology of puberty. 1. Normal sexual maturation. J Pediatr 1973;83:1–19. Illustrations from Fleisher GR, Ludwig S. Textbook of pediatric emergency medicine. 2nd ed. Baltimore: Williams & Wilkins, 1988:1205.

Timing of Normal Pubertal Development in Females (For females in the United States, the entire sequence is displaced to the left by 4 to 6 months.)

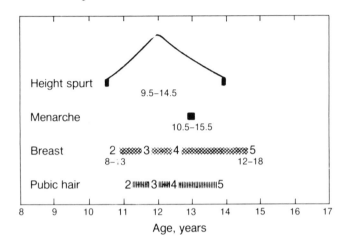

Timing of Normal Pubertal Development in Males[a]

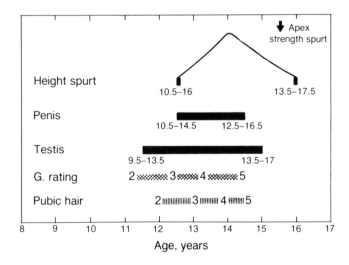

[a]Adapted with permission from Tanner JM. Growth and endocrinology of the adolescent. In: Gardner LI, ed. Endocrinology and genetic diseases of childhood and adolescents. 2nd ed. Philadelphia: W.B. Saunders Co. 1975:20,31.

Denver II

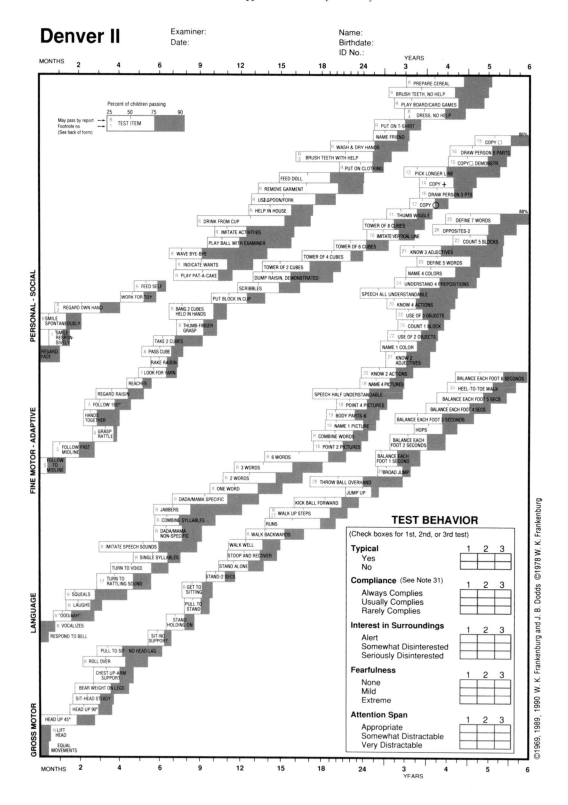

Denver II

Examiner:
Date:

Name:
Birthdate:
ID No.:

DIRECTIONS FOR ADMINISTRATION

1. Try to get child to smile by smiling, talking or waving. Do not touch him/her.
2. Child must stare at hand several seconds.
3. Parent may help guide toothbrush and put toothpaste on brush.
4. Child does not have to be able to tie shoes or button/zip in the back.
5. Move yarn slowly in an arc from one side to the other, about 8" above child's face.
6. Pass if child grasps rattle when it is touched to the backs or tips of fingers.
7. Pass if child tries to see where yarn went. Yarn should be dropped quickly from sight from tester's hand without arm movement.
8. Child must transfer cube from hand to hand without help of body, mouth, or table.
9. Pass if child picks up raisin with any part of thumb and finger.
10. Line can vary only 30 degrees or less from tester's line.
11. Make a fist with thumb pointing upward and wiggle only the thumb. Pass if child imitates and does not move any fingers other than the thumb.

12. Pass any enclosed form. Fail continuous round motions.
13. Which line is longer? (Not bigger.) Turn paper upside down and repeat. (pass 3 of 3 or 5 of 6)
14. Pass any lines crossing near midpoint.
15. Have child copy first. If failed, demonstrate.

When giving items 12, 14, and 15, do not name the forms. Do not demonstrate 12 and 14.

16. When scoring, each pair (2 arms, 2 legs, etc.) counts as one part.
17. Place one cube in cup and shake gently near child's ear, but out of sight. Repeat for other ear.
18. Point to picture and have child name it. (No credit is given for sounds only.)
   If less than 4 pictures are named correctly, have child point to picture as each is named by tester.

 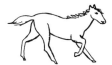

19. Using doll, tell child: Show me the nose, eyes, ears, mouth, hands, feet, tummy, hair. Pass 6 of 8.
20. Using pictures, ask child: Which one flies?... says meow?... talks?... barks?... gallops? Pass 2 of 5, 4 of 5.
21. Ask child: What do you do when you are cold?... tired?... hungry? Pass 2 of 3, 3 of 3.
22. Ask child: What do you do with a cup? What is a chair used for? What is a pencil used for? Action words must be included in answers.
23. Pass if child correctly places and says how many blocks are on paper. (1, 5).
24. Tell child: Put block **on** table; **under** table; **in front of** me, **behind** me. Pass 4 of 4. (Do not help child by pointing, moving head or eyes.)
25. Ask child: What is a ball?... lake?... desk?... house?... banana?... curtain?... fence?... ceiling? Pass if defined in terms of use, shape, what it is made of, or general category (such as banana is fruit, not just yellow). Pass 5 of 8, 7 of 8.
26. Ask child: If a horse is big, a mouse is __? If fire is hot, ice is __? If the sun shines during the day, the moon shines during the __? Pass 2 of 3.
27. Child may use wall or rail only, not person. May not crawl.
28. Child must throw ball overhand 3 feet to within arm's reach of tester.
29. Child must perform standing broad jump over width of test sheet (8 1/2 inches).
30. Tell child to walk forward, 👣👣👣 ➤ heel within 1 inch of toe. Tester may demonstrate. Child must walk 4 consecutive steps.
31. In the second year, half of normal children are non-compliant.

OBSERVATIONS:

Reproduced with permission from Frankenburg WK, Dodds J, Archer P, Shapiro H, Bresnick B. The Denver II: a major revision and restandardization of the Denver developmental screening test. Pediatrics 1992;89:91–97.

References and Additional Readings

Pediatric History, Physical Exam, and Approach to the Pediatric Patient:

Algranati PS. Pediatric clinical encounter. In: Willms JL, Lewis J, eds. Introduction to clinical medicine. Media, Pennsylvania: Harwal, 1991.

American Academy of Pediatrics Committee on Psychosocial Aspects of Child and Family Health. Guidelines for health supervision. 2nd ed. Elk Grove Village, Illinois: American Academy of Pediatrics, 1988.

Athreya BH, Silverman BK. Pediatric physical diagnosis. Norwalk, Connecticut: Appleton-Century-Crofts, 1985.

Barness LA. Manual of pediatric physical diagnosis. 5th ed. Chicago: Yearbook Medical Publishers, Inc., 1981.

Boyle Jr. WE, Hoekelman RA. The pediatric history. In: Hoekelman RA ed. Primary pediatric care. St. Louis, Missouri: C.V. Mosby, 1987:52–62.

Dworkin PH, Wible KL, Sutherland MC, Humphrey N. Manual of pediatric anticipatory guidance. Morgantown, West Virginia: Department of Pediatrics, W. Virginia University Medical Center, 1986.

Gundy JH. The pediatric physical examination. In: Hoekelman RA, ed. Primary pediatric care. St. Louis, Missouri: C.V. Mosby, 1987:63–109.

Hoekelman RA. The physical examination of infants and children. In: Bates B. A guide to physical examination and history taking. 4th ed. Philadelphia: J.B. Lippincott Co., 1987:525–598.

Simms MD. Pediatric ambulatory care center well-child care forms and guide. Waterbury, Connecticut: St. Mary's Hospital, 1988.

Solomon R. Pediatric experiences in year II clinical sciences. E. Lansing, Michigan: Department of Pediatrics and Human Development, College of Human Medicine, Michigan State University, 1986.

Telzrow RW. Anticipatory guidance in pediatric practice. J Cont Educ Pediatr 1978;20:14–27.

Adolescent:

Copeland KC. Variations in normal sexual development. Pediatr Rev 1986;8:18–25.

Emans SJH, Goldstein DP. Pediatric and adolescent gynecology. 2nd ed. Boston: Little Brown and Co., 1982.

Goldenring JM, Cohen E. Getting into adolescent heads. Contemp Pediatr 1988;July:75–90.

Hofmann AD, Greydanus DE. Adolescent medicine. 2nd ed. Norwalk, Connecticut: Appleton & Lange, 1989.

Newborn:

Klaus MH, Fanaroff AA. Care of the high risk neonate. 3rd ed. Philadelphia: W.B. Saunders, 1986.

Specialties:

American Academy of Pediatrics Committee on Infectious Diseases. Report of the committee on infectious diseases. 21st ed. Elk Grove Village, Illinois: American Academy of Pediatrics, 1988.

Frankenburg WK, Dodds J, Archer P, Shapiro H, Breswick B. The Denver II: a major revision and restandardization of the Denver Developmental Screening Test. Pediatrics 1992;89:91–97.

Hurwitz S. Clinical pediatric dermatology. Philadelphia: W.B. Saunders, 1981.

Jones KL. Smith's recognizable patterns of human malformations. 4th ed. Philadelphia: W.B. Saunders, 1988.

Nelson LB. Pediatric ophthalmology. Philadelphia: W.B. Saunders, 1984.

Renshaw TS. Pediatric orthopedics. Philadelphia: W.B. Saunders Co., 1986.

General Pediatric Texts/Review Books:

Behrman RE, Vaughan III VC, Nelson WE, eds. Nelson textbook of pediatrics. 13th ed. Philadelphia: W.B. Saunders, 1987.

Dworkin PH, ed. The national medical series for independent study: pediatrics. New York: John Wiley & Sons, Inc., 1987.

Rudolph AM, Hoffman JIE, eds. Pediatrics. 18th ed. Norwalk, Connecticut: Appleton & Lange, 1987.

Useful Lists and Hard to Locate Clinical Information:

McMillan JA, Nieburg PI, Oski FA. The whole pediatrician catalogue, Vol 1, Philadelphia: W.B. Saunders Co., 1977.

McMillan JA, Stockman JA, Oski FA. The whole pediatrician catalogue, Vol 2, Philadelphia: W.B. Saunders Co., 1979.

McMillan JA, Stockman JA, Oski FA. The whole pediatrician catalogue, Vol 3, Philadelphia: W.B. Saunders Co., 1982.

Index